HEALTH AND SOCIETY
SERIES
General Editor
NORMAN KREITMAN

Alcohol and Illness

The Epidemiological Viewpoint

WITHDRAWN

edited by

JOHN C. DUFFY

EDINBURGH UNIVERSITY PRESS

© Edinburgh University Press 1992

Edinburgh University Press
22 George Square, Edinburgh

Typeset in Lasercomp Palatino
by Alden Multimedia Ltd, Northampton and
printed in Great Britain at The Alden Press, Oxford

A CIP record for this book is available from
the British Library.

ISBN 0 7486 0353 0

Contents

The Contributors

GEOFFREY R. COHEN   Lecturer, Department of Mathematics and Statistics, University of Edinburgh.

JOHN C. DUFFY   Senior Lecturer, Department of Mathematics and Statistics, University of Edinburgh, on secondment to Alcohol Research Group, Department of Psychiatry, University of Edinburgh.

STEPHEN W. DUFFY   Non-clinical Scientist, Medical Research Council Bio-statistics Unit, Cambridge.

GILLIAN M. RAAB   Lecturer, Medical Statistics Unit, Department of Public Health Sciences, University of Edinburgh.

LINDA D. SHARPLES   Non-clinical Scientist, Medical Research Council Bio-statistics Unit, Cambridge.

E. JAN WATERSON   Lecturer, Department of Applied Social Studies and Social Work, University of Keele.

Foreword

This book brings together a collection of papers, specially written for this volume, on the major health risks known or suspected to be associated with drinking. The approach is mainly epidemiological, that is, based on studies of human populations, rather than, for example, laboratory studies of animals. Where appropriate, the authors evaluate the strength of the evidence to date relating alcohol to the medical conditions considered, in terms of quality of study design, control of other variables and consistency of findings across studies. For the most part, the papers are quite technically sophisticated, using currently available statistical methods to compare studies in more detail than previously. The source materials used comprise the major research studies in each field available at the time of editing (September 1991), and hence the book also serves as a useful reference source. What it does not do, however, is present opinions as definitive conclusions. Where controversy exists regarding the causal role of alcohol in the illnesses considered, the evidence is presented, and in some cases an opinion expressed, but without any claim of finally resolving the issues.

The papers relate to questions involving the level of understanding of the phenomena considered, the quality of research, and in particular cases the consensus medical opinion concerning the possible causal role of alcohol consumption. Where possible, risks associated with consumption at various levels are estimated and put into a public health context by examining the possible impact of alcohol on population mortality and morbidity by cause. For this purpose, most chapters use the population of England and Wales rather than Scotland, and there are two reasons for this. The first is that the former population is ten times larger than that of Scotland, which makes for increased stability in rates over time, especially for rare phenomena. Secondly, much more extensive and recent survey information concerning population alcohol consumption is available for England and Wales. The years chosen to illustrate population aspects are recent, but are not identical in all papers, reflecting the times at which the work was begun.

A brief description of epidemiological and statistical methods is given in the first chapter to aid interpretation of the rest of the book. Readers completely unfamiliar with the application of statistics may prefer to skip Chapter 1, but Section 1.8 will be helpful in understanding why it is that epidemiological studies rarely yield definitive results, and why scientific controversy in this area is so common.

Finally, it must be emphasised that the papers do not attempt to deal directly with alcoholism or social problems due to alcohol, alcohol-related crime and alcohol-related accidents, but focus entirely on health and illness.

John C Duffy
Edinburgh
30 September 1991

1 The Epidemiology of Risk Assessment

In considering the relationship between alcohol consumption and various forms of physical health damage, we may distinguish two possible approaches. One, the experimental approach, would essentially involve administering alcohol in controlled amounts to a group of animals in a laboratory and comparing the subsequent development of illness in these animals with that in a group of animals not exposed to alcohol. This might be further complicated by having several groups of animals, each receiving different amounts of alcohol. Assuming the assignment of animals to groups was carried out by a randomisation procedure, the results of such experimentation could be used to determine the possible causal role of alcohol consumption in the development of illness in animals. Extrapolation of these results to human beings would be controversial, and although studies of the effects of alcohol on animal health are performed and reported, this book concentrates on epidemiological studies of the association between alcohol consumption and ill health in human populations. It will be useful then to give some account of what epidemiology is, and the nature and limitations of the most commonly used epidemiological methods.

Modern epidemiology developed from the study of epidemics of infectious disease, although nowadays epidemiological methods are also employed in the study of non-infectious disease. Epidemiological studies are based on the idea of observing population processes, rather than intervening directly in individual cases, other than perhaps as part of a general diagnostic or screening procedure. So, while most people are familiar with the experimental method in science, in which researchers manipulate aspects of the environment and observe the consequences of such manipulation, this is not the approach of epidemiology. The reasons for this relate to feasibility, and moral and ethical questions. It is clearly immoral to experiment on individuals with possibly harmful substances to assess whether they are harmful or not. Epidemiologists have neither the desire nor the opportunity to assign people randomly to exposure to possibly dangerous environmental, chemical, nutritional or other agents.

Epidemiology is thus essentially an observational science. In infectious disease, epidemiology has played an important part in understanding the processes leading to diseases such as cholera, poliomyelitis and tuberculosis and in demonstrating the causal role of rubella in early pregnancy in the production of congenital defects, and has led to the construction and application of successful preventive strategies. In non-infectious disease, such as various forms of cancer, epidemiological methods have successfully identified risk factors such as cigarette-smoking, asbestos and others. Nevertheless, epidemiological methods cannot be as stringent as experimental methods, and the observation of an association between a possible risk factor and an illness by epidemiological methods falls far short of demonstrating that the risk factor plays a causal role in the development of the illness. In order to understand the epidemiological approach and its limitations, it is useful to describe some of the main tools of investigation employed in the various studies which are reviewed later in this book, and to explain the statistical methods which are used to draw conclusions from them.

Several types of study design are in common use in epidemiology. Each type involves the collection and analysis of counted data, such as frequencies of occurrence of events, numbers of individuals having particular attributes and so on. To make this more concrete, we might consider an event to be the development of a particular illness, and the attribute as being a total abstainer or a drinker. We might then compare the numbers of drinkers developing the illness with the number of abstainers doing so. Of course, in such a comparison, we would need to take into account the numbers of drinkers and abstainers actually studied, in order to determine an appropriate rate of development of illness for each group.

1.1 General population studies

One possible method of investigating the association between exposure to a possible risk factor and the occurrence of an illness is to select a random group of individuals from the population for investigation. In a cross-sectional study, the individuals are assessed for the presence or absence of the illness in question and a number of potential risk factors at the time of the investigation. If the respondents are followed up over a period of time subsequent to the start of the study, we call the design a longitudinal or prospective study. In studies of this kind, the outcome of interest may simply be the total number of individuals with the illness at the end of the study, or the time taken for each individual to develop the illness. The latter approach is not discussed here, as this method is not used in the studies to be reviewed later.

If we follow up a random sample from the appropriate population, there is one basic statistical quantity or parameter which it seems natural to estimate, and that is the incidence rate of the illness. This is defined simply as the number of individuals developing the illness divided by the total number of individuals in the study. An annual incidence rate may be calculated by dividing this rate by the time period of the study in years, and it is usual to express rates as rates per 100,000 or per 1,000,000, which

Table 1.1: Two-way classification of respondents

		Disease		
		Present	Absent	TOTAL
Risk	Present	a	b	m_1
Factor	Absent	c	d	m_2
	TOTAL	n_1	n_2	n

requires multiplication by the appropriate constant. Rates should be corrected if individuals leave the study, through, for example, death or cessation of cooperation. The denominator after correction is then person-years at risk.

In a cross-sectional study, it is only possible to calculate a so-called prevalence rate, which is simply the number of individuals suffering from the illness at the time of the study divided by the total number in the study. This poses certain difficulties, as prevalence relates to incidence in a rather complicated fashion, involving factors such as duration of illness, time to death, and incidence of cure. Nevertheless, prevalence may be analysed by the same methods as incidence, but care is needed in the interpretation of such analyses. Rothman (1988, pp. 32–4) provides a useful discussion of these issues.

The purpose of the prospective study is to examine the effect of possible risk factors on the development of disease. We might classify individuals in a prospective study according to whether they exhibit a particular attribute (the potential risk factor), and whether they develop the disease. We may then estimate incidence rates for those with and without the attribute.

Table 1.1 shows how the information from such a classification might be presented. Entries in the table are frequencies corresponding to each category. It is important to notice that the only quantity in the table which is fixed in advance is the total number of individuals in the study, n. Clearly, the population rate of illness may be estimated as n_1/n, and the rates in the risk factor present and absent groups as a/m_1 and c/m_2 respectively. Unless n is particularly small, the significance of the difference between these two rates may be assessed by means of the usual χ^2 test for a two by two contingency table applied to the data in Table 1.1, or equivalently a test of the difference between two proportions. However, the difference between the two rates is not usually the measure of choice in epidemiology for describing the association between risk factor exposure and disease. There are a number of reasons for this, and we shall see later that some common types of epidemiological study do not permit estimation of this rate difference. Two measures in common use are the relative risk and the odds ratio.

1.2 *Relative measures of disease incidence*

The relative risk of disease associated with a particular risk factor is defined as the ratio of the rate among those exposed to the factor to the rate among the unexposed. In the notation of Table 1.1, the relative risk is estimated by

$$\hat{rr} = \frac{a/m_1}{c/m_2} \tag{1.2.1}$$

This quantity measures how much more or less likely it is that disease occurs among those exposed to the factor in question. It takes values between zero and infinity, and represents positive or negative association accordingly as rr is greater than or less than one respectively. Notice that in the latter case the factor, rather than being a risk factor, may be a protective factor for the illness in question.

The odds ratio, usually denoted ψ, is another common measure of association. The probability of an event e, p say, can be re-expressed in terms of odds, O(e), as follows:

$$O(e) = \frac{p}{1 - p} \tag{1.2.2}$$

Thus, given the rates of illness, which may be considered as probabilities of illness, we may calculate the odds for the exposed and unexposed groups. In terms of the quantities in table 1.1, the odds ratio ψ may be estimated as

$$\hat{\psi} = \frac{ad}{bc} \tag{1.2.3}$$

The most attractive feature of the odds ratio as a measure of association is that it may be estimated in situations where neither the rate difference nor the relative risk can, as we shall see in the next sections. Another useful aspect is that it approximates the relative risk quite well if the incidence rate of the disease is small. To see this, consider an illness with rates r_e and r_u among the exposed and unexposed members of the population. The relative risk is then

$$rr = \frac{r_e}{r_u} \tag{1.2.4}$$

and the odds ratio is

$$\frac{r_e(1 - r_u)}{r_u(1 - r_e)} \tag{1.2.5}$$

If r_u and r_e are both small, then the quotient of the two bracketed terms is approximately equal to 1.

Table 1.2: Deaths in a ten-year study of English civil servants

		Outcome		
		Death	Survival	TOTAL
Alcohol	Abstainer	45	432	477
Consumption	Drinker	68	877	945
	TOTAL	113	1,309	1,422

As an example of a prospective study, consider the following data from a longitudinal study of English civil servants (Marmot et al., 1981). The outcome of interest is death during the ten years of the study, and the table classifies the individuals as abstainers or drinkers. In the original study, these data were presented in a more detailed classification (see Chapters 3 and 6).

From Table 1.2, we can easily calculate the ten-year death rates as 0.0943 among the non-drinkers and 0.0720 among the drinkers. The estimate of relative risk is thus 1.31 considering the non-drinkers as the exposed category. The odds ratio estimate is 1.34, showing a reasonably close approximation to the relative risk. This analysis is undertaken purely for illustrative purposes, and the data will be considered in more detail later.

1.3 Cohort studies

Another way of assessing the association between a possible risk factor and illness is to follow two groups of individuals over time, with one group exposed to the factor in question and the other not exposed. The results of such a study can be tabulated and analysed by the methods of the previous section, but there is one difference worth noting. The population proportions exposed to the risk factor could be estimated from the general population study, but in a cohort study the numbers of individuals in the exposed and unexposed groups, m_1 and m_2 in the notation of Table 1.1, are determined by the experimenter.

Nevertheless, rates of illness among the exposed and unexposed groups may be estimated from cohort studies, and an estimate of relative risk obtained directly. This is not so for the next type of study design to be considered.

1.4 Case-control studies

In a case-control study, sometimes called a retrospective study, the researcher compares a group of individuals with the illness in question (cases) with a group free from the illness (controls). The numbers in the groups are determined by the investigator, so studies of this type do not permit estimation of the rates of illness among the exposed or unexposed groups. To see this, consider the results of such a study in the form of Table 1.1.

Table 1.3: Smoking and cataract in Edinburgh

	Cataract Cases	Population Controls	Total
Smoker	298	87	385
Non-smoker	569	236	805
Total	867	323	1,190

The totals n_1 and n_2 are chosen by the investigator, and different choices of these will lead to different values of a/m_1 and c/m_2. It follows that these cannot be estimates of the true rates among the exposed and unexposed, and hence the relative risk cannot be estimated (Cornfield, 1951). Knowledge of the population rate of illness is required in order to estimate the relative risk from a case-control study, and for many conditions such information is not available. However, the odds ratio is estimable from such a study, and the estimate is just as in the previous case:

$$\hat{\psi} = \frac{ad}{bc} \qquad (1.4.1)$$

The rationale of the estimate is slightly different. Essentially, the argument is that the frequencies should be weighted to take account of the different sampling fractions for cases and controls, which would imply multiplying the entries in the disease present (case) column by a constant, X say, and the entries in the disease absent (control) column by Y. The odds for the exposed group may be estimated as the ratio of cases to controls in the exposed category, and similarly for the unexposed. This implies that each set of odds, is weighted by the same constant, X/Y. On taking the ratio of the two odds, the constant cancels, giving the result. Another way of looking at this is to consider risk factor prevalence among the case and controls. If we let p_1 and p_2 be the proportions of cases and controls respectively with the risk factor, then it follows that our estimates of these would be a/n_1 and b/n_2 in the notation of Table 1.1. Our estimates of the complementary probabilities, q_1 and q_2, are similarly c/n_1 and d/n_2. Thus the odds ratio may be expressed in terms of risk factor prevalences as $p_1 q_2 / p_2 q_1$.

The data in Table 1.3 are taken from a case-control study of cataract in Edinburgh (Clayton et al., 1980). Notice that the population rate of cataract is certainly not 867/1190, these numbers being simply the sizes of the case and control groups. However, the odds ratio for cataract due to smoking is estimable as

$$\hat{\psi} = \left(\frac{298^*236}{87^*569} \right) = 1.42 \qquad (1.4.2)$$

The usual χ^2 test gives a value of 5.95 on 1 degree of freedom indicating strong evidence of association, between smoking and cataract.

Table 1.4: Example of matched case control study

	Risk Factor	Control Present	Absent	Total
	Present	a	b	m_1
Case	Absent	c	d	m_2
	Total	n_1	n_2	n

1.5 Matched case-control studies

Apart from the risk factor under investigation, other variables such as age, sex and unknown risk factors may affect the probability of developing illness, and may also be associated with presence of the risk factor. Such variables are said to be *confounding*, and one way to take account of known confounding factors is by individually matching each case to a control who shares the potentially confounding characteristics of the case. The resulting study design, the matched case-control study, is rather different from the previous types considered, and data analysis is different also.

The entries in Table 1.4 are the frequencies of case-control *pairs* classified according to the presence or absence of the risk factor for each member of the pair. Thus for example there are b pairs in which the case member has the risk factor and the control does not. The total in the table, n, is simply the total number of pairs, which is of course one half the total number of individuals involved.

It is obvious that rates cannot be estimated directly from the data in Table 1.4, and it might appear that the odds ratio will also pose problems of estimation. However, the odds ratio is in fact estimated very easily as

$$\hat{\psi} = \frac{b}{c} \tag{1.5.1}$$

This may be shown by considering the probabilities p_1 and p_2 that a case and a control are positive on risk factor exposure.

Defining
$$q_1 = 1 - p_1 \tag{1.5.2}$$

and
$$q_2 = 1 - p_2 \tag{1.5.3}$$

it follows that the probability that a discordant pair has the case member of the pair being exposed to the risk factor, and the control member not is given by

$$\left(\frac{p_1 q_2}{p_1 q_2 + q_1 p_2} \right) \tag{1.5.4}$$

Similarly, the probability of a discordant pair being such that the case member does not have the risk factor while the control member does is

$$\left(\frac{p_2 q_1}{p_1 q_2 + q_1 p_2} \right) \tag{1.5.5}$$

Hence the estimate in equation (1.5.1) is the maximum likelihood estimate of the odds ratio, as the observed proportions are maximum likelihood estimates of the appropriate probabilities. Notice that pairs which are not discordant do not contribute to the estimation procedure, nor to statistical testing. The test used in these circumstances is a binomial test that the probability of each type of discordant pair is 0.5, given the total number of discordant pairs, which for large values of b+c may be performed by means of a χ^2 test on 1 degree of freedom. This procedure is often called McNemar's test.

1.6 The logistic-linear model

An alternative method of analysing studies of these types, and one which as we shall see lends itself to more complicated analyses of higher dimensional tables, is provided by logistic regression, which is widely implemented in computer packages such as GLIM (Payne, 1985).

The model postulates a linear regression of log-odds of illness risk on values of the exposure variable. For the exposed population, the appropriate quantity is $\log(r_e/(1-r_e))$, and for the unexposed, $\log(r_u/(1-r_u))$, in the notation of Section 1.2. Notice that the difference of these two *logits* is simply $\log\psi$. Now consider a regression equation in which the dependent variable, y, is the logit of the rate of illness, and the independent variable, x, is exposure at levels 0 (corresponding to no exposure) and 1 (corresponding to exposure). The regression equation may be written

$$E[y] = \alpha + \beta x \qquad (1.6.1)$$

so for the unexposed group the model gives

$$\log(r_u/(1 - r_u)) = \alpha \qquad (1.6.2)$$

and for the exposed group

$$\log(r_e/(1 - r_e)) = \alpha + \beta \qquad (1.6.3)$$

Hence the parameter β in the model corresponds to the logarithm of the odds ratio due to exposure. Estimation of β and its standard error will permit point and interval estimation of the odds ratio, in addition to testing the significance of the effect of exposure.

With the case-control study, matters are not so clear-cut. The difficulty here is, as before, that the proportion of cases in a particular exposure category is not an estimate of the rate in that category. However, the argument can be extended to cover the case-control situation as follows.

In the simple case of one exposure variable, we may express the conditional probability of illness given exposure as

$$P(c/e) = \frac{P(e/c)P(c)}{P(e)} \qquad (1.6.4)$$

where c denotes the event 'illness' and e exposure. This relation implies that the probabilities which are estimable from the case-control study, namely the conditional probabilities of exposure, given illness (for the cases), and absence of illness (for the controls) are related to the probabilities of illness given exposure or absence of exposure by multiplication by the appropriate constants. It is easy to see that these constants cancel in the odds ratio as before. In order for this argument to be valid, it is essential that the probability that an individual, whether a case or control, is selected is independent of exposure status, and that the selection process is independent for different individuals.

Although we have not yet considered the multivariate case in detail, it is convenient to express the argument in terms of a vector of exposure variables, $\mathbf{x}$. From a theoretical point of view, a difficulty is posed by the undeniable fact that in a case-control study it is the exposure status of individuals, $\mathbf{x}$, which is a random variable, not their case status, which is controlled by the selection procedure. Denoting case or control status by y, and exposure status by $\mathbf{x}$, we can write

$$P(\mathbf{x}/y) = \frac{P(y/\mathbf{x})P(\mathbf{x})}{P(y)}; \quad y = 0,1 \qquad (1.6.5)$$

where P(y) corresponds to the probability of case (1) or non-case (0) status. The case-control study provides information about $P(\mathbf{x}/y)$, which is $P(y/\mathbf{x})$, multiplied for cases by the overall probability of exposure divided by the probability of illness, and for controls by the probability of exposure divided by the probability of not having the illness. The logistic-linear model for $P(y/\mathbf{x})$ appears therefore to require modification for application to case-control studies. However, if the marginal distribution of exposure does not contain information about the parameters of the model for $P(y/\mathbf{x})$ then it is possible to estimate $P(\mathbf{x})$ and the coefficients of the model jointly. This joint likelihood approach leads to the same parameter estimates as applying the logistic linear model directly to the data.

An appropriate alternative is to use conditional likelihood methods to eliminate the term in $P(\mathbf{x})$. This is based on application of the logistic linear model conditional on the x_i values observed in the case and control groups in terms of their randomisation distribution. The method leads to computational difficulties for large sample sizes, and asymptotically the resulting estimates will be close to those obtained by the joint likelihood method. A fuller theoretical treatment of these issues is provided by Farewell (1979).

The logistic-linear model may be further generalised to include explanatory variables reflecting exposure to several categories of the risk factor. In the case of ordered multiple exposure categories with m levels, $x_1, x_2, ..., x_m$, we may fit $m-1$ constants to the levels 2, 3, ... m and such an independent variable would be called a factor. An alternative approach is to fit a single regression coefficient β, and in this model we will refer to x as a variate. The models for these are as follows, with y representing the logit of the appropriate proportion:

$$E[y/x_k] = \alpha + \beta_k; k = 2, 3, \ldots m \qquad (1.6.6)$$

$$E[y/x] = \alpha + \beta x \qquad (1.6.7)$$

These are simply extended to vectors of independent variables, which may include both factors and variates. Polynomial terms may be fitted by creating new variates having the values of the appropriate powers of the variates concerned.

1.7 Use and interpretation of logistic linear models

Suppose we have observed n values y_i, i = 1, 2, ... n. Corresponding to each of these is a vector of p explanatory variables x_i. For a linear model, the systematic component is

$$E[y_i] = \alpha + \sum_{j=1}^{p} \beta_j x_{ij} \qquad (1.7.1)$$

where α is called the intercept, and the regression coefficients are the β_js. Note that some or all of the explanatory variables may be dummy variables constructed to represent different levels of a factor. In the case of the logistic linear model, the y_is are proportions corresponding to the various categories in the table of data, and the random component in the model arises from the binomial distribution with parameters p given by $E[y_i]$, and n_i, the appropriate marginal total.

If we fitted n linearly independent parameters β_i, then the maximum likelihood estimate (mle) of $E[y_i]$ would be equal to y_i/n_i, and the results of the fit would be perfect. This is called the saturated model. On the other hand, suppose we attempt to fit a single constant to all the y_is. In this case, the mle of y_i is α for all i. This is referred to as the null model, and somewhere in between these two extremes we hope to find a model which both explains and simplifies the data.

For any model, we can obtain the corresponding value of the likelihood function, evaluated at the point where it is maximised. Suppose the likelihood for a particular model, m say, is ℓ_m, and the likelihood for the saturated model is ℓ_s. Then a statistical test of whether m is a satisfactory model may be obtained using the scaled deviance statistic,

$$S(m,s) = -2\log\left(\frac{\ell_m}{\ell_s}\right) \qquad (1.7.2)$$

Large values of this statistic indicate lack of fit of the model, and statistical significance may be assessed by comparing with the χ^2 distribution, with degrees of freedom given by the difference in the number of parameters in the two models.

In general, to compare any two models, one of which is nested under the

Table 1.5: Ascitic cirrhoses and controls by daily alcohol consumption

Daily consumption (in gms 100% alc)	Ascitic Cirrhosis Patients	Population Controls
0–20	3	185
21–40	10	212
41–60	15	165
61–80	24	108
81–100	30	58
101–120	23	31
121–140	25	13
141–160	24	5
161+	30	1

other, in the sense that the more complicated or larger model contains all the parameters present in the smaller, the deviance difference between the two models provides a test of significance of the terms in the larger model not present in the smaller. The smaller model differs from the larger in that some of the parameters in the latter are set to zero in the smaller model. Statistical testing as above using the χ^2 distribution essentially tests the null hypothesis that the true values of these parameters are zero.

As an example, consider the data in Table 1.5 which are taken from a study of liver cirrhosis and alcohol consumption in Ille et Vilaine (Pequignot et al., 1978).

Table 1.5 represents the distributions by alcohol consumption category of 184 male sufferers from alcoholic cirrhosis and 778 male controls obtained from the general population. The nine consumption categories may be considered as nine levels of a single factor, or we may associate with each category a value of consumption. For example, the first category may be taken to correspond to 10 gms/day, the second 30 gms/day, and so on. There is clearly some arbitrariness in this procedure, which is particularly evident when considering the last category, which has no upper limit. Nevertheless, it is a useful exercise to investigate the feasibility of replacing the eight degrees of freedom factor with a single degree of freedom variate. The success or failure of the simpler (variate) formulation may be assessed by comparison of the deviance differences between the models with the appropriate percentage point of χ^2 on 7df. However, in the present case, fitting alcohol consumption as a factor at nine levels will result in a residual deviance of zero, with zero degrees of freedom, and we may therefore perform a single analysis with a suitably defined variate. First, however, it is necessary to assess whether there is any association at all between consumption and risk of liver cirrhosis, and this may be done by fitting the null model, that is a single constant to all the proportions.

The resulting scaled deviance is 327.34 on eight degrees of freedom, which is highly statistically significant on comparison with the χ^2 distribution. We may therefore conclude that there is an association between consumption and cirrhosis risk, and proceed to fit alcohol consumption as an explanatory variate. We assign values 10, 30, 50, ..., 170 to represent consumption in each of the categories, and fitting this variate yields a residual scaled deviance of 3.43 on seven degrees of freedom. This is clearly much less than the 5% point of the appropriate χ^2 distribution, and we conclude that the differences in risk between the categories may indeed be adequately modelled by a logistic regression on the values of consumption. Another way of interpreting this result is to view the residual deviance after fitting consumption as a variate as providing a test of non-linearity in the logistic relationship between consumption and risk. The non-significant value of the deviance indicates that there is no evidence of non-linearity in the relationship.

The estimated regression coefficient is 0.039, with a standard error of 0.0028, and this may be interpreted as indicating that if alcohol really is causal, and not simply associated with cirrhosis risk as a result of some unmeasured relationships or processes, an increase of one gram of alcohol in daily consumption increases the log-odds ratio of cirrhosis by 0.039. To put this in a more concrete way, a person drinking an extra 20 grams of absolute alcohol per day multiplies his odds ratio of cirrhosis by approximately $e^{0.39}$, or 2.2, and for low values of initial risk this is approximately equivalent to risk multiplication by the same factor.

There is some arbitrariness in the choice of 170 gms per day to represent the highest consumption category, since it is open-ended. Notice however that different but sensible values chosen to represent the maximal consumption category produce roughly similar values of the deviance and the estimated regression coefficient.

1.8 Bias, confounding and causality

As mentioned earlier, there is a large gap to be bridged between establishing an association between a risk factor and disease, and demonstrating a causal relationship. Among the possible reasons why an association might exist in the absence of causation are bias and confounding.

For the purposes of illustration, we will consider a case-control study with a single risk factor which may be present or absent. Selection bias occurs when for one reason or another the criteria for admission into the control group differ from those for entry to the case group. An obvious example of this is self-selection, when for example the control group is recruited from volunteers who are aware of the subject of study. In an epidemiological study of cataract in Edinburgh (Clayton et al., 1980), some controls were recruited by newspaper advertisement for volunteers. As there was an interest in possible genetic factors, information was recorded as to the numbers of relatives with cataracts. The volunteer controls turned out to have more in-laws with cataract than did the cases. However, rather than interpreting this as showing that the absence of cataract among in-laws is a risk factor for cataract, it is more likely that the result was due to bias. The implication is that volunteers with a wife or husband suffering from cataract had decided to join the study precisely because they wished to assist in a study of this subject.

A related form of selection bias results from the so-called 'healthy worker' effect. It is generally found that the mortality experience of the working population is less than that of the population as a whole. Although it may sometimes be convenient to select controls from a group of workers in a hospital for example, this is likely to introduce bias.

Another type of bias may arise from the increased likelihood of cases being diagnosed from the population with the possible risk factor than from the population without the factor. For example, suppose it is believed, but not demonstrated, that alcohol consumption predisposes to a particular illness which is difficult to diagnose unequivocally. In making the diagnosis of the illness, the physician may be influenced towards a positive finding by the drinking status of the patient. A subsequent case-control study using these cases will show an association between the factor and illness which may be entirely due to the respondents' alcohol consumption having influenced the diagnosis before the study began.

Confounding arises in epidemiological studies from the causal intervention in a relationship under study of an uncontrolled extraneous variable. Although it may also be a problem in experimental research, it poses particular difficulties in epidemiology, because of the lack of opportunity to assign individuals randomly to study groups to be compared. As an example, consider an epidemiological investigation to assess the relative risk rr of developing an illness due to exposure to E. An extraneous variable X could obscure or exaggerate the relation between illness and exposure if it is associated with E and also with the probability of developing the illness. It is even possible that the direction of the true relationship between E and X could be reversed due to confounding. A particularly clear instance of a potential confounder is smoking habits in studies relating alcohol consumption to health. Smoking is known to be positively associated with the development of serious illnesses, and also with alcohol consumption. Hence if smoking habits are not controlled for, alcohol consumption will appear to be associated with these illnesses.

There is an interesting result concerning the relative risk of illness due to X if X is entirely responsible for an observed association between E and illness, measured as a relative risk rr. The relative risk due to exposure to X must be at least as strong as that apparently due to exposure to E, and in addition X must be rr times more common among those exposed to E as in those unexposed. Taken together, these two conditions are often considered to be good reasons for using relative risk as the measure of choice for relative disease incidence, large values of relative risk being unlikely to be due entirely to an unidentified confounding variable.

Potentially confounding variables may be controlled for in the statistical analysis of the results of a study, and there are several aspects of this which could be discussed at length. A particularly important consideration is that of course only measured variables can be controlled for. The effects of potential confounding variables which have not been measured as part of the study cannot be controlled. A second point is that it is important in reporting the results of controlling for confounders to provide values of the estimates of association after adjustment. It is not enough simply to report that an association remains significant after adjustment.

It may seem incongruous after the discussion above that causal inferences are ever made on the basis of epidemiological studies, but there are some general guidelines which provide a degree of reassurance concerning causal interpretations of observed associations. It is well to keep in mind that while it is theoretically impossible to 'prove' the causal nature of an association, as Hill (1965) writes,

> All scientific work is incomplete – whether it be observational or experimental. All scientific work is likely to be upset or modified by advancing knowledge. That does not confer upon us a freedom to ignore the knowledge we already have, or to postpone the action that it appears to demand at a given time.

Of the many rules of thumb seeking to provide a basis for causal inferences in epidemiology, four of particular importance are strength of association, dose-response, the temporal relation between risk and exposure, and consistency across different studies.

The main reason for interpreting a strong association between a possible risk factor and disease as unlikely to be due to confounding relates to the result concerning relative risk mentioned earlier. The confounding variable would have to be at least as strongly associated with risk as the factor under investigation, and the association of this confounding variable with the factor would also have to be of this magnitude. Hence it is argued that such a confounder would be unlikely to go unrecognised. Similar considerations rule out the possibility of bias being responsible for the observed association. On the other hand, it does not necessarily follow that no weak associations are causal in origin, but clearly in such cases other arguments need to be applied to support the notion of causality.

A dose-response relationship also increases confidence in causal inference. The strength of a causal association would be expected to increase with increasing levels and duration of exposure to the risk factor. It is nevertheless possible for dose-response-type relationships to be due to confounding, and it is not always the case that a causal agent should necessarily produce higher risk of illness with higher levels of exposure.

In terms of temporal relationship, it is clear that a cause must be antecedent to an effect. More particularly, for some types of cancer quite detailed information has been gathered about latency periods. If the temporal relationship between the possible risk factor and disease is inconsistent with known temporal aspects of the development of the illness, then an observed association is unlikely to be causal.

Finally, the demonstration of similar associations in different populations in various circumstances lends support to causal interpretation, although differences in methodology may lead to differences in the observed magnitudes of associations.

For further discussion of causality, bias, confounding and methods of controlling for possibly confounding variables, see Breslow and Day (1980, Ch. III) and Rothman (1986, pp. 16–20, 82–90).

1.9 Comparing results from several studies and calculating attributable risks

It is generally the case that studies relating a particular risk factor to a disease are carried out by different groups of researchers in different countries at various times. When data are available from the studies concerned in similar forms, it is usually quite simple to compare and, if appropriate, combine their results. In particular, the logistic linear model may be employed, with an extra explanatory variable which identifies the study from which the data were obtained. This variable, which should be considered as a factor with number of levels corresponding to the number of studies involved, will always be fitted in the logistic-linear model, but is usually of limited interest. If the results are all from longitudinal studies, differences between levels of the study factor will simply reflect differences in length of follow-up periods and base-rates. When some case-control studies are included in the data under analysis, study factor estimates will reflect differences in the design and control proportions used.

Of considerably more interest are the terms in the model corresponding to risk-factor exposure, and the interaction between study and exposure. If the latter term is statistically significant, then for some reason or another there exist significant differences in the relationship between exposure and risk in the different studies. In these circumstances, it is not desirable to attempt to provide a combined risk estimate (or set of estimates in the case of a risk factor at several levels) from the studies concerned, although for practical purposes it may be necessary to do so. It is however possible to conclude that the factor under investigation is associated with the disease if all the odds-ratio estimates are in the same positive direction. If the interaction between study and exposure is not statistically significant, then all the studies are essentially telling the same story about the relationship between the risk factor and the disease, and it is then quite legitimate to produce a single estimate.

Of course, in many cases data will not be available from the studies concerned in a suitable form for such combined analysis. Nevertheless, if odds-ratio estimates are available, it is possible to assess whether they show significant differences between studies, and then to produce a combined estimate if appropriate. Rather than detail the statistical methodology here, the interested reader is referred to Breslow and Day (1980, pp. 139, 142–3).

Considering now the question of estimating the importance from a public health point of view of a particular risk factor in terms of the proportion of disease accounted for by exposure to the factor, let us suppose that we have determined a value of the relative risk, w, for mortality from a particular cause in the simplest case, with a single cause of death and a binary (present/absent) risk factor. (The same approach may be taken to the estimation of morbidity.) The attributable risk estimate represents the percentage reduction in mortality which would follow removal of the risk factor from the population. In particular, let it be supposed that the rates of death from the cause in question are respectively r and wr among the non-exposed and the exposed. Further suppose that the proportion of the population exposed to the risk factor is p, while the complementary proportion $(1-p)$ is not exposed.

It follows that the population death rate is $pwr+(1-p)r$, while if the risk factor could be removed the death rate would be simply r. The excess mortality due to the risk factor is then given by the population size times the difference between these rates, $rp(w-1)$, while the attributable risk percentage is given by

$$\frac{100p(w - 1)}{p(w - 1) + 1} \qquad (1.9.1)$$

In order to estimate this quantity, it is necessary to estimate w, the relative risk due to exposure, and p, the proportion of the population exposed. It is worth emphasising that the value of attributable risk depends on the proportion of individuals in the population exposed to the risk factor. For this reason, it is not appropriate to apply an attributable risk estimate made in one population to a different population. To estimate attributable mortality, or numbers of deaths, it is also necessary to estimate either the existing population rate of death or the rate among the unexposed. Moreover, for the attributable risk estimate to bear interpretation as the expected percentage reduction in mortality, it is necessary that the risk factor actually be so − that is that the relation between mortality and exposure be causal, and not due simply to confounding for example.

The concept of attributable risk may be extended to categorical and continuous risk factors, at the expense of complicating the algebra slightly as follows:

Suppose the risk factor is a categorical variable with $k+1$ categories, $i = 0, 1, 2, ..., k$, where category 0 represents the absence of the factor in question. We write the relative risks in categories 1 to k with respect to category 0 as w_1, w_2, ... w_k, and the death rate in category 0 as r. Let the population proportions in the various categories be denoted p_0, p_1, ..., p_k. Then, by the above argument the population rate will be given by

$$p_0 r + r \sum_1^k p_k w_k \qquad (1.9.2)$$

If the entire population were free from the risk factor, the population rate would be r. Hence the attributable risk percentage due to the risk factor is given by

$$\frac{100\left(p_0 + \sum_1^k p_k w_k - 1\right)}{p_0 + \sum_1^k p_k w_k} \qquad (1.9.3)$$

By a similar argument, we may extend the notion to a protective factor, in which case the appropriate index is referred to as the prevented fraction.

In dealing with a continuous risk factor, we may estimate the effect of a reduction of the level of exposure throughout the population using the logistic regression coefficients. The method is somewhat arbitrary, but likely to be valid for rare conditions. The logistic regression model has

$$\text{logit}(p) = \alpha + \beta x \qquad (1.9.4)$$

where p is the probability of mortality, α is an unidentifiable intercept, x is the value of the risk factor and β is the estimated regression coefficient. If the present average value of the risk factor in the group at risk is x, the above is the formula for logit probability of mortality in that group. If we now consider the same group in other respects except with x replaced by 0.5x, we have

$$\text{logit}(p') = \alpha + 0.5\beta x. \qquad (1.9.5)$$

where p' is the probability corresponding to the new value of the risk factor. The log relative risk is estimated by the log-odds ratio, i.e.

$$-0.5\beta x. \qquad (1.9.6)$$

The exponential of this is the relative risk, and multiplying the existing rate by this quantity provides an estimate of the expected new rate for the population with values of the risk factor halved.

References

Breslow, N.E. and Day, N.E. (1980) *Statistical Methods in Cancer Research Volume 1*, Lyon: International Agency for Research on Cancer.

Clayton, R.M., Cuthbert, J., Phillips, C.I., Bartholomew, R.S., Stokoe, N.L., Ffytche, T., Reid, J.McK., Duffy, J., Seth, J. and Alexander, M. (1980) Analysis of individual cataract patients and their lenses – a progress report, *Experimental Eye Research* 31: 553–66.

John C. Duffy

Farewell, V.T (1979) Some results on the estimation of logistic models based on retro-
    spective data, *Biometrika* 66: 27–32.
Hill, A.B. (1965) The environment and disease: association or causation, *Proceedings of the
    Royal Society of Medicine* 58: 295–300.
Marmot, M.G., Shipley, M.J., Rose, G. and Thomas, B.J. (1981) *Alcohol and mortality − a
    U-shaped curve, Lancet* 14 March: 580–3.
Payne, C.D. (ed.) (1985) *The GLIM System Release 3.77 − Manual*, Oxford: NAg Ltd.
Pequignot, G., Tuyns, A.J. and Berta, J.L. (1978) Ascitic cirrhosis in relation to alcohol
    consumption, *International Journal of Epidemiology* 7: 113–20.
Rothman, K.J. (1986) *Modern Epidemiology*, Boston: Little, Brown and Co.

2 The Measurement of Alcohol Consumption

To use epidemiological methods to study the possible influence of alcohol consumption as a risk factor for disease, it is necessary to develop some way of obtaining information from respondents concerning their drinking habits. This is not as simple a matter as it might at first seem, as has been discovered in the field of general population surveys. Later chapters in this book will use survey data to provide estimates of the proportions of the population in various alcohol consumption categories for the calculation of attributable risk along the lines of equation (1.9.3), and it is therefore appropriate to consider measurement of consumption in surveys and in epidemiological research together.

A question not often addressed directly in studies of the relationship between alcohol consumption and health is the nature of the possible link, and its implications for measurement. In many societies and cultures, the drinking habits of individuals change over their lifetimes, sometimes in association with changes in their social and family responsibilities, or, for example, experience of health problems which need not be related directly to alcohol consumption. Hence the current drinking habits of an individual may only be a rough guide to his or her overall lifetime consumption of alcohol, which is implicitly the relevant aspect of exposure in terms of risk of chronic disease. The problems of measuring contemporary consumption are difficult enough, and this may be one factor deterring researchers from attempting to elicit lifetime consumption.

2.1 Units of measurement

The scale of measurement of alcohol consumption by individuals poses the first problem. Respondents may typically drink several different types of beverage, each of which will have a specific concentration of alcohol. The volume of beverage drunk may be fairly standard, particularly if purchased and consumed in retail premises such as bars, public houses, restaurants and so on, but this will not necessarily be the case with consumption at home, at parties or in other private settings.

Respondents' consumption is therefore ascertained in terms of drinks of various sizes of various beverages, and is then converted into alcohol at 100%, either in terms of volume or weight. Of course, the results of such conversion are approximations, as most beverages, even of the same general type, will vary considerably in terms of their alcohol content. In the usual approach to measurement, respondents report their consumption under the headings of beer, wine, fortified wine and spirits, and a standard conversion factor is applied to the total in each category. In more sophisticated approaches, beer may be subdivided into 'normal strength' and high strength, and wine into red and white, with different conversions being applied in these subcategories. In surveys in the United Kingdom, measurements are transformed to units of alcohol, one unit being approximately equivalent to half a pint of beer, a single measure of spirits, a glass of wine or a glass of fortified wine. Considerable care may be taken to measure home consumption accurately, required because of the absence of a standard amount served. Wilson (1981) describes the use of drinking glasses and measuring jars by interviewers in eliciting home consumption. In the epidemiological literature, it is possible to find measurements in terms of 'drinks', grams of alcohol, fluid ounces of alcohol, centilitres of alcohol and units. The final estimate of individual consumption remains rough and ready whatever method is used, although many studies give the illusory appearance of accuracy in measurement.

It is well known in sample surveys in general that different forms of what is essentially the same question may produce different results, both in terms of participation in the survey and in the actual responses to the question (Kalton and Schuman, 1982), and this has been documented in the field of alcohol surveys by Poikolainen and Karkkainen (1985). Even with the 'best' question-wording possible, alcohol surveys may suffer from deliberate concealment, forgetting and problems in contacting heavy drinkers. Concealment may occur both in epidemiological studies and population surveys because the respondent considers his or her own drinking to be excessive or stigmatising, while in population surveys in which respondents are contacted at domestic addresses it may be difficult to find heavy drinkers at home. Various methods of obtaining information from respondents have been adopted, for example, drinking diaries (Poikolainen and Karkkainen, 1983), self-completion questionnaires and computer interviewing (Waterton and Duffy, 1984), but in most epidemiological applications and national surveys direct face-to-face interviewing is used. In general it is estimated that survey estimates of total population consumption constitute from 40% to 60% of consumption known to take place from official sources such as taxation records. As a result, the 'success' of a measurement method is often judged simply by the amount of consumption elicited – the higher the admitted consumption, the better the method (Midanik, 1982).

2.2 Individual alcohol consumption

In any population survey or epidemiological study, the complex nature of drinking behaviour also gives rise to problems of measurement. Respondents differ in the types of beverage they drink, the amounts of each beverage they drink on occasions of drinking, and their frequency of drinking. Within individual considerations raise further complications. The same person drinking the same beverage on different occasions may drink different amounts, while in consecutive weeks an individual may undertake different numbers of drinking occasions which may involve the use of different beverages.

When assessing the various methods in use to measure alcohol consumption, it is important to bear in mind that in epidemiological research the most important aspect is the classification of respondents by individual levels of consumption. This is necessary in order to examine the relationship between individual experience of disease and consumption, and, in the population, is essential to calculation of attributable risk. Disaggregation of consumption and aspects of consumption by subpopulations defined by criteria other than consumption level will also be required. For example, many studies of mortality relate to specific sex and age groups. In order to calculate attributable risks, the distribution of consumption within similarly-constructed groups will require to be estimated.

2.3 Quantity—Frequency measurement

The Quantity—Frequency (Q–F) Index introduced by Strauss and Bacon (1953) represents an early attempt to obtain information about drinking behaviour from survey respondents. Typically, respondents are asked about their drinking of each of three types of alcoholic beverage, namely beers, wines and spirits. For each beverage type, the usual frequency of drinking that beverage is recorded on a list ranging from 'three or more times a day' to 'never'. The usual quantity of each beverage type drunk on each occasion of drinking that beverage is also elicited.

In order to take account of variability in respondents' drinking habits, the index was modified to the Quantity—Frequency—Variability Index described by Cahalan and Cisin (1968). This involved altering the questions relating to the quantities of each beverage as follows: for each beverage type which the respondent claimed to drink once a month or more frequently, the proportions of occasions on which five or more, three or four and one or two units were drunk were obtained by questioning, the available replies being 'nearly every time', 'more than half the time', 'once in a while' or 'never'. A further question concerning the frequency of drinking of any alcoholic beverage was also asked, and categorisation proceeded on the basis of the reply to this question, together with the modal and maximum quantities of the most frequently consumed beverages.

The Volume—Variability Index was introduced by Cahalan and Cisin (1968) and attempted to classify each respondent by his average daily volume of consumption and, within several groups of particular daily volumes, to subclassify by the day-to-day variability of the respondents. The average daily volume was estimated by multiplying the frequency of consumption (expressed as drinking occasions per thirty days) by the modal amount of each beverage.

The response categories for Q–F-based questions may be further elaborated, for example more recent practice in respect of determining the proportion of occasions on which various amounts of each beverage are consumed would use a wider scale of proportions and an increased number of amount categories.

Although this method is widely used, there are some difficulties with its interpretation in terms of rate of consumption. First, it is not clear how respondents interpret the questions, which certainly seem to be requiring the report of modal rather than average frequencies and quantities. If the within-individual (temporal) distributions of these measurements are positively skew, then the averages will often be greater than the modes. Some indirect evidence on this question may be obtained from surveys using a different measurement approach, in that when respondents are asked about the typicality of their reported consumption in the week before interview, the majority reporting untypical consumption assert that drinking in that week was more than usual. See for example Goddard and Ikin (1988), Table 3.2.

A second difficulty concerns possible question-wording and response-category effects. Practical experimentation could lead to improved question-wording and a fuller understanding of respondents' interpretation of the questions. Response-category effects in this area are well known and discussed by Bradburn and Sudman (1982). Their conclusion is that these effects are best allowed for by providing very high response categories.

Finally, a technical problem arises. If the averaging procedures implicitly used by the respondent in answering the questions relate to different time periods for establishing frequencies and amounts, then some degree of bias will result in converting these responses to a rate of consumption.

2.4 Description of occasions

Several approaches to measurement are based on the description of drinking occasions by the respondent. Of these, the most frequently encountered is based on consumption by the respondent in the week prior to interview. 'Last week's consumption' has for several years now been standard practice in UK surveys. Respondents are asked to provide detailed information about consumption on each drinking occasion in the last week, starting with the day immediately before the interview, and then covering each of the preceding six days in reverse temporal order. Interviewers are normally instructed to provide memory prompts to respondents who appear uncertain as to their activities on any particular day. Often supplementary questions about a longer period of past time are asked of respondents who report no consumption in the week before interview.

This methodology is generally thought to decrease possible memory

problems, and to allow less scope for question wording effects by mini-
mising individual interpretation of questions. Restricting attention to last
week's consumption produces a low yield of information concerning those
individuals who drink infrequently. However, in epidemiological studies of
the association between alcohol-related problems and the rate of alcohol
consumption, lack of information concerning infrequent drinkers (who will
generally have a low rate of consumption) may not be a disadvantage.

A more important difficulty relates to variability of individual consumption. If week-to-week variation in the amount of alcohol consumed is
relatively large, then the ordering of individuals by reported consumption
using this method will not reflect their ordering over a longer time period.
This will have the effect of obscuring links between consumption and
variables associated with it. In particular, the apparent risk in the consumption categories relative to the zero consumption category will be biased in
the direction of unity; that is, if consumption increases risk, the effect
estimate will be underestimated, whereas for a protective effect the relative
risk will be overestimated.

While it is relatively simple and speedy to enquire about respondents'
behaviour over the past week day by day, and to provide memory prompts,
this obviously represents a formidable task over a longer time period. In
fact, some studies (e.g. Marmot et al., 1981) use recall of consumption over
a period shorter than one week, with a consequent increase in potential
attenuation and underestimation of relationships.

2.5 Implications

The under-reporting of consumption by individuals, known to occur in
population surveys, has considerable implications for epidemiological
studies of alcohol and illness. If, as seems likely, under-reporting also occurs
in assessment of alcohol consumption in epidemiology, then relationships
between consumption and risk of harm will be 'too steep'. The risk increase
apparently corresponding to a particular amount of alcohol will in fact
correspond to a greater amount. Thus, if a particular level of risk increase
obtained from epidemiological study is used to set a 'safe' limit or threshold,
the apparent limit will be lower than the actual quantity of alcohol corresponding to the risk increase. To put this another way, a particular level of
risk established from an epidemiological study is associated not so much
with *consuming* a particular amount of alcohol, but with *reporting* the
consumption of that amount.

In reconciling epidemiological studies with population data, for example
in the calculation of attributable risk, it is important that methods of
measuring consumption should be as similar as possible. Consider an
epidemiological study which used a quantity–frequency approach to
measurement, and subsequently converted the respondents' values to units
per week. In applying the results of the study to a population for the

calculation of attributable risk, it will be advisable to use an estimate of the distribution of consumption in the population obtained by a quantity–frequency approach, rather than a 'last week's consumption' method.

Measurement differences will affect the comparison of results from different studies. Differences in response bias or under-reporting between studies, as might be expected when analysing studies from different cultures, will lead to different estimates of the parameters of the dose-response relationship, and this may appear as a significant interaction between study and consumption in statistical analysis. Although Q–F measurement may be difficult to interpret in terms of the behaviour of the respondents, it is less likely to be affected by within-individual temporal variation than measurement of last week's consumption, and so should produce a more stable ordering of individuals by their consumption level, with less misclassification. Hence a difference in dose-response estimates is to be expected between studies using different measurement methods in cultures showing appreciable temporal variation in individual drinking.

Finally, it is important to bear in mind when interpreting the results of epidemiological studies relating alcohol consumption to risk of illness that many of these studies were designed for the investigation of other risk factors; for a discussion of this topic in general, see Feinstein (1988). Consequently, little attention may have been paid to the measurement of consumption, and in some cases reports of the studies will not contain a clear description of the methods used, which may bear little relation to good practice and knowledge in this area. As a result, their conclusions should be treated with some caution, particularly as regards dose-response relationships and thresholds of harm.

References

Bradburn, N.M. and Sudman, S. (1982) *Asking Questions*, San Francisco: Jossey-Bass.

Cahalan, D. and Cisin, I.H. (1968) American drinking practices: summary of findings from a national probability sample. Vol. I: Extent of drinking by population subgroups, *Quarterly Journal of Studies on Alcohol* 29: 130–51.

Feinstein, A.R. (1988) Scientific standards in epidemiologic studies of the menace of everyday life, *Science* 242: 1257–63.

Goddard, E. and Ikin, C. (1988) *Drinking in England and Wales in 1987*, London: HMSO.

Kalton, G. and Schuman, H. (1982) The effect of the question on survey responses: a review, *Journal of the Royal Statistical Society* 145: 42–75.

Marmot, M.G., Shipley, M.J., Rose, G. and Thomas, B.J. (1981) *Alcohol and mortality – a U-shaped curve*, *Lancet* 14 March: 580–3.

Midanik, L. (1982) The validity of self-reported alcohol consumption and alcohol problems: a literature review, *British Journal of Addiction* 77: 357–82.

Poikolainen, K. and Karkkainen, P. (1983) Diary gives more accurate information about alcohol consumption than questionnaire, *Drug and Alcohol Dependence* 11: 209–16.

Poikolainen, K. and Karkkainen, P. (1985) Nature of questionnaire options affects estimates of alcohol intake, *Journal of Studies on Alcohol* 46: 219–22.

Strauss, R. and Bacon, S.D. (1953) *Drinking in College*, New Haven: Yale University Press.

Waterton, J.J. and Duffy, J.C. (1984) A comparison of computer interviewing techniques and traditional methods in the collection of self-report alcohol consumption data in a field survey, *International Statistical Review* 52: 173–82.

Wilson, P. (1981) Improving the reliability of drinking surveys, *The Statistician* 30: 159–67.

3   Alcohol and All-cause Mortality

There have been several recent attempts to estimate the proportion of deaths from all causes in England and Wales which may be attributed to the consumption of alcohol. A number of different methodological approaches have been adopted for this purpose, each of which pose specific difficulties. This chapter will review past work briefly, and consider in detail the data used in one approach to the problem. Together with more recent British data these show that a statistical approach based on studies of total mortality as a function of alcohol consumption is not sufficient to resolve the problems.

3.1 Alcohol and mortality

The consumption of alcohol is known to be a risk factor for liver cirrhosis, accidental death and certain types of malignancy, as well as being a direct cause of death by poisoning. However, as will be seen in later chapters, the possible causal role of alcohol in illnesses accounting for the major proportion of total mortality is still at an early stage of investigation. The position is further complicated by the continuous nature of alcohol consumption and by the resulting need to estimate not just a single value of relative risk but a dose-response relationship. There is also the question of deciding what is to be considered as the dose or level of exposure — lifetime consumption or current consumption? More controversially, the possibility that alcohol consumption may offer some protection against risk of death from cardiovascular disease could lead to a 'credit ' side of the mortality account.

McDonnell and Maynard (1985) attempted to estimate mortality attributable to alcohol consumption by considering for each of a number of diagnoses an exposed 'alcoholic' category, estimating mortality among alcoholics and non-alcoholics, and calculating the excess mortality on the basis of the proportion of alcoholics in the population, along the lines of Equation (1.9.1). Deaths from each diagnostic category were then summed to give the total mortality attributable to alcohol. However, this method ignores alcohol-related excess mortality among non-alcoholic members of the population and, more problematically, requires estimation of the prevalence of alcoholism. The 'high' estimate of the proportion of alcoholics used by these authors was based on a methodology now discredited (Schmidt and de Lint, 1970). Given that the estimate being derived is really the proportion of deaths due to alcoholism rather than alcohol consumption, it is reasonable to omit consideration of a possible protective effect of light to moderate consumption.

The Royal College of Physicians (1987) estimated the proportion of deaths due to alcohol consumption on the basis of a study carried out among Swedish men aged between 46 and 48 (Petersson et al., 1982). The Swedish investigators judged 25% of deaths among these men to be alcohol-related, and this figure was applied to mortality in England and Wales. No attempt was made to estimate risk parameters or risk factor prevalence. Different patterns of illness, mortality, alcohol consumption and particularly exposure to other risk factors between Sweden and the United Kingdom would require to be taken into account in any methodologically sound application of the Swedish results to England and Wales.

An approach similar to that of McDonnell and Maynard is evident in the estimate produced by the Royal College of General Practitioners (1986). Again, a number of different causes of death are analysed separately and attributable mortality is estimated. However, the basis of this estimation is in general far from clear, and certainly cannot accord with attributable risk estimation, since the references cited do not in general provide sufficient information to permit estimation of the attributable risk of mortality due to alcohol. They either report associations between alcohol and deaths from various causes without controlling for other risk factors, notably smoking, or are simply earlier guesstimates of the proportions of deaths from various causes due to alcohol. An exception is the paper by Rothman (1980) on malignant neoplasm mortality, in that the author makes an attempt to quantify the influence of alcohol on cancer mortality in the United States, considering various causes and cancers of different sites. His conclusion is that about 3% of all cancer mortality in the US is due to alcohol, and the figure used in the RCGP report is consistent with this. However, the report does not consider the differences in the mix of cancer mortality between the United Kingdom and the United States, and the proportions of deaths from different types of cancer are central to Rothman's work.

None of the references cited in respect of the various causes of deaths provide scientifically derived estimates of the proportion of mortality attributable to alcohol. While most would agree that the majority of deaths from liver cirrhosis and chronic liver disease are indeed due to alcohol, the position is much less clear for other causes of death. The link between alcohol consumption and death by accident is in particular cases easy to discern, but on a population basis McDonnell and Maynard gave a 'high' estimate of the proportion of road accident deaths due to alcohol as 40%. This makes the RCGP report's estimate that 40% of *all* fatal injuries and poisonings are due to alcohol high indeed.

3.2 Direct study of mortality

Anderson (1988) adopts a different approach to the problem. Although he implicitly uses the notion of attributable risk, in his work he considers data concerning mortality from all causes classified by alcohol consumption category from a number of studies. Alcohol consumption is analysed as a categorical risk factor, and estimated risks are calculated for each category. The population distribution of alcohol consumption in England and Wales obtained by survey methods (Wilson, 1980) is then used to estimate the proportion of the population in each of the categories, and attributable mortality estimated. It should be noticed that Anderson does not calculate attributable mortality due to alcohol as such, but, since he chooses to use the light drinking category as his baseline, it is mortality due to consumption of over ten units per week that is being estimated. Had he chosen to use the zero consumption category as the reference, then the result in almost every study considered would have been that alcohol consumption would appear to be responsible not for *excess* mortality but for *diminished* mortality.

Anderson is rightly critical of the methodology used in earlier studies attempting to estimate the impact of alcohol on mortality. However, he is less forthcoming about the problems inherent in his own approach, and surprisingly misses some methodological deficiencies of his five basic sources. For convenient reference, these are listed here:

The Honolulu Heart Study (HHS) (Blackwelder et al., 1980)
The UK male civil servants (Whitehall) study (WS) (Marmot et al., 1981)
The Kaiser-Permanente study (KPS) (Klatsky et al., 1981)
The Chicago Western Electric study (CWES) (Dyer et al., 1980)
The Framingham Study (FS) (Gordon and Kannel, 1984)

Anderson seeks to assess the numbers of deaths from all causes in the UK which may be attributed to alcohol, on the basis of risk estimates for all-cause mortality from these five studies. A major difficulty is that four of the five relate to the United States, and there are several problems of applying rates or relative risks from one population to a different population. For simplicity, we consider mortality from a single cause first, and then go on to show how all-cause mortality poses even greater difficulties.

The death rate for a single cause of death in one country will in general reflect the distribution of risk factors in that country, which may include specific genetic factors peculiar to the population. When rates are calculated by subgroups of the population, as for example in the case of groups consuming different amounts of alcohol, these will also reflect the distribution of other risk factors within the subgroups. If these other risk factors are associated with consumption categories, they will act to bias estimates of the association between consumption and mortality. Considering a similar categorisation of a different population, there are several reasons to expect the subgroup rates to be different. First, it is obvious that the overall death rate from the cause under consideration is very likely to differ between the countries, for reasons which may be related to other risk factors and differences in the age structure of the populations. If these are associated with consumption, then the estimates of the subgroup rates will be inappropriate, and so will be the rate ratios or relative risks (which are implicitly the quantities used by Anderson, although his explanation is in terms of rates). Secondly, it is quite possible that for genetic or environmental reasons one population might be more or less susceptible to the cause of death than the other, and this may lead to a difference in association between the factor under investigation and mortality. There are several further points which could be made, particularly differences in the associations between consumption and confounders in the two populations, but it is perhaps more useful now to discuss all-cause mortality in the light of the above.

Suppose now that, contrary to the above speculations, the relationships between consumption and individual causes of mortality in terms of relative risks are indeed the same in the two populations. In that case, it will be appropriate to calculate excess mortality from a single cause in the second population from the relative risks estimated from the first. However, it will definitely not be appropriate to proceed in this way when considering all-cause mortality, for the following reason. It is well known that alcohol consumption is associated with different causes of mortality in different ways. For example, a U-shaped relation between alcohol consumption and mortality from heart disease has been extensively reported, whereas the relation between alcohol consumption and liver cirrhosis mortality appears to be of the more usual sigmoid type. Unless the proportions of deaths from each single cause in the all-cause figures are the same in the two populations, these differences in relationships between individual causes will ensure that the all-cause relationship differs between the two populations. As will be seen later, statistical analysis supports these caveats and indicates that differences of these natures do appear to be of importance.

A further difficulty relates to the classifications of drinkers employed in the five source studies. None of these uses the same methods of measurement as Wilson's population survey, and this poses a serious problem of validity, as discussed in Chapter 2. The matching of categories from the source studies to those used in Wilson's published table is even more peculiar. For example, the lowest consumption band in the Whitehall study is identified by Anderson with 1–10 units per week. It is clear from the original paper that this band corresponds in fact to 1–7 of Wilson's units per week. Similar difficulties and inaccuracies arise in connection with his consideration of the US studies, which variously report measurements in terms of drinks, ounces and millilitres. Had these problems been recognised, the data reported by Wilson would have permitted estimation of the England and Wales population proportions in the various categories by interpolation. The analysis presented later addresses the issue of categorisation by first of all attempting to convert the categories in the published sources to units of alcohol per week, and then using class midpoints to reflect the appropriate consumption level. Nevertheless, no claim is made here of *compatibility* in the methods of measurement.

The age and sex structures of respondents are also a source of difficulty. Most of the studies concern only middle-aged men, and it may be quite inappropriate to extrapolate attributable risk estimates calculated from a study of 40 to 55-year-old men to an entire population. The study from which Anderson obtained his final estimates, the KPS, appears not to suffer from this problem, in that both male and female adult respondents were included. However, there is a deficiency in using overall results rather than age-specific findings from this study, caused by differences in age structure between the study population in the San Francisco Bay area and the England and Wales population.

In fact, the Kaiser-Permanente study turns out to be the least useful of the five considered, because of its matched design. From the published description of the study, it appears that the groups were constructed by individual matching on selected characteristics to individuals in the highest consumption category. One important consequence of this is that the lower consumption groups are extremely unlikely to be representative of the general population members consuming at the same level, and it is inappropriate to apply rates derived from these groups even to the population of the geographical area providing the subjects of the study, far less the population of England and Wales. As mentioned in Chapter 1, ratios of marginal rates are not good estimates of relative risk in matched studies (Breslow and Day, 1980).

3.3 Statistical analyses

That the above difficulties have real impact on the relation between alcohol and mortality can be demonstrated by statistical analysis of the datasets used by Anderson, supplemented for interest by further mortality data from the British Regional Heart Study (BRHS) reported by Shaper et al. (1988), and from the American Cancer Society study (ACSS) (Boffetta and Garfinkel, 1990). Table 3.1 shows the mortality data used, with alcohol consumption for each category estimated as the midpoint of the appropriate interval, except in the case of the highest (open) intervals, where 'reasonable' values have been estimated. In every case, the figures used are unadjusted for other risk factors such as smoking habits and age. The denominators for the ACSS study were obtained by dividing person-years at risk in Table 2 of the published work by the length of follow-up period. The category 'irregular drinker' from this study is not included in the

Table 3.1: Mortality by alcohol consumption category

Study	Alcohol consumption	Number of deaths	Number at risk
HHS	0	264	3,747
	4	66	1,316
	14	86	1,583
	35	93	1,232
WS	0	45	477
	4	24	390
	18	24	367
	40	20	189
CWES	0	13	77
	3	83	555
	10	77	542
	24	66	428
	44	25	152
	70	32	78
FS	0	155	402
	4	179	668
	11	66	264
	17	45	175
	30	104	344
	50	51	131
	75	46	122
BRHS	0	41	466
	0.5	142	1,845
	8	143	2,544
	30	116	2,042
	55	62	832
ACSS	0	23,147	136,734
	3	2,683	16,700
	10	4,509	30,332
	20	3,684	21,304
	30	1,933	10,105
	40	1,343	6,532
	50	688	2,989
	70	1,775	6,709

analysis, due to the difficulty of estimating a value of consumption for this group. The analyses reported represent an approach to exploring the differences and similarities between the studies, and should not be treated as definitive, although it is difficult to see how any major improvement in methodology might be effected on the basis of available data, and if it could be, that it would have much impact on the conclusions of the present analysis.

The data were analysed by means of the GLIM computer package (Payne, 1985), considering the numbers of deaths in each category as a

Table 3.2: Model deviances and test statistics in analysing mortality

Model	Residual Deviance	Degrees of Freedom	Difference	Degrees of Freedom
Null Fit	2,573.30	33		
Full Model	138.60	16	2,435.0	17
Excluding Interactions	175.95	26	37.35	10

binomial response variate, with the numbers at risk forming the binomial total. A code for study was fitted as a factor at six levels, and alcohol consumption was fitted as a variate, together with the square of alcohol consumption to take account of a possibly quadratic relationship. Fitting study as a factor adjusts for possibly different overall mortality rates between the studies, which arise naturally from different lengths of follow-up period, as well as age structure and other differences between the populations on which the studies were based.

Of crucial interest for the estimation of attributable mortality is that the relationship between alcohol consumption and mortality be roughly the same in all studies. This may be tested by fitting terms representing the interaction of study with alcohol consumption, both linear and quadratic, and examining their magnitude and statistical significance. The appropriate test statistic is the difference in residual deviance between the model including the interaction terms and that with these terms omitted. The results of model fitting are presented in Table 3.2. The full model deviance shows lack of fit, implying that taking all the studies together there may be other aspects of the dose-response relation than the linear and quadratic which merit investigation.

The test statistic for the significance of the interaction terms is 37.35 on 10 degrees of freedom, which may be compared with the χ^2 distribution, and is significant at the 0.1% level. Thus the studies do indeed indicate differences in the relationship between alcohol and mortality in the different study populations. These may be examined further by considering the effect estimates for the linear and quadratic terms relating alcohol to mortality, but for conciseness we consider here a further analysis relating to the two British studies.

3.4 Attributable risk analysis based on the British studies

Analysing only the Whitehall study and the British Regional Heart study data, the linear and quadratic components of consumption reduce the residual deviance by 10.0 on 2 degrees of freedom, to a value of 9.6 on 5 degrees of freedom, showing a satisfactory fit. We may therefore estimate relative risks based on the combined data from these studies. To calculate attributable risk estimates, population data regarding consumption may be

Table 3.3: Calculation of attributable risk using BRHS categories and population consumption data from Goddard and Ikin (1988)

Consumption category	Relative Risk (RR)	Population Proportion (p)	RR times p
Abstainer	1.00	0.06	0.06
Occasional (<1 unit/wk)	1.00	0.20	0.20
Light (1–15 units/wk)	0.86	0.50	0.43
Moderate (16–42 units/wk)	0.75	0.19	0.14
Heavy (>42 units/wk)	1.09	0.05	0.05
Total			0.88

estimated from the OPCS survey reported by Goddard and Ikin (1988). In their report, Table 2.13 gives alcohol consumption data for men over 25 in ten-year bands. The Whitehall study subjects were aged between 40 and 64, and the BRHS subjects from 40 to 59. Thus the Goddard and Ikin bands do not correspond exactly to either of these studies, and it was decided to use information regarding men aged between 45 and 64. BRHS categories were employed because they are more detailed than those used in the Whitehall study. The consumption categories reported in Goddard and Ikin are different from those in BRHS, and the appropriate population proportions were therefore estimated from the tabulation by piecewise linear interpolation on a log-probability plot. Table 3.3 shows the results of this analysis.

Taking for granted the caveats mentioned above, the analysis shows that the death rate among men aged between 45 and 64 in 1987 is estimated to be 0.88 of the value it would be if they all were abstainers. In other words, it could be said that assuming the relation between alcohol and mortality to be directly causal, alcohol consumption in the population, far from being a cause of excess mortality, is in fact a protective factor. In fact, there were 55,045 deaths among men aged from 45 to 64 in 1987. This is 0.88 of the number of deaths that would be expected if the death rate for abstainers applied to the entire population. Thus we may calculate an expected number of deaths if the abstainer rate applied as 62,551, indicating that alcohol consumption by the population led to there being 7,506 *fewer* deaths than would have occurred had the entire population been abstinent.

3.5 Implications

It might appear from the above that while statistical objections to the use of North American studies to estimate the association between alcohol and mortality appear well founded, the British studies could be used for this purpose. Nevertheless, there are a number of difficulties associated with such a procedure, not all theoretical. First, it is clear that using the zero consumption category as baseline, alcohol consumption acts as a protective factor to reduce rather than increase mortality. However, so far as cardio-vascular mortality — the major cause of death in both the British studies — is concerned, there is evidence to suggest that at least some of this apparent protection may be due to ill subjects changing their drinking habits (Shaper et al., 1988). Although the general U-shaped relation between alcohol consumption and mortality has been found to persist in some populations after excluding the already ill (Room and Day, 1974), Shaper et al. found no such persistence in the BRHS population, the relationship found at aggregate level deriving from that section of the study population who had previous cardiovascular diagnoses. It therefore remains a matter for further investigation in the UK as to whether consumption exerts a protective influence on mortality among the already ill.

To some extent the data available to Shaper could be used to investigate his hypotheses more fully. Instead of using grouped logistic regression, it is possible to perform a case-by-case analysis, taking as explanatory variates alcohol consumption, age, class, smoking and burden of illness. Such an analysis would establish whether this burden of illness model is sufficient to explain the persistence of the apparent protective effect of alcohol consumption among those men with an initial recall of diagnosis.

If Shaper's explanation is correct, and the apparent protective effect of alcohol is due to those most at risk of mortality reducing their consumption, we are led to the conclusion that studies of total mortality will not provide satisfactory estimates of mortality due to alcohol consumption. Shaper's figures show that in his group of over 5,800 men who reported no recall of doctor diagnosis, there is no significant relationship between consumption and mortality. This should not, however, be interpreted as implying that the net effect of alcohol consumption on mortality is zero. Mortality in a given time period is a relatively rare phenomenon, and the bulk of such mortality in middle-aged men in the United Kingdom is accounted for by cardiovascular and cardiovascular-related conditions, together with various types of cancer. If alcohol consumption is not related to *these* conditions, then it will appear unrelated to *total* mortality except in very large samples indeed.

In the absence of any final resolution of the controversy over the protective effect of alcohol consumption, attempts to calculate the numbers of deaths from all causes due to alcohol are doomed to failure in scientific terms, even if they might be successful from a public relations point of view (see, for example, Humphris et al., 1991). What would be justifiable would be estimation on the basis of such data as are available of the contribution of alcohol to deaths from particular causes, such as liver cirrhosis, certain forms of cancer, and so on. However, in interpreting the resulting estimates, the possibility of compensating or more than compensating protective effects cannot yet be dismissed.

References

Anderson, P. (1988) Excess mortality associated with alcohol consumption, *British Medical Journal* 297: 824–6.

Blackwelder, W.C., Yano, K., Rhoads, G.G., Kagan, A., Gordon, T. and Palesch, Y. (1980) Alcohol and mortality: the Honolulu heart study, *American Journal of Medicine* 68: 164–9.

Boffetta, P. and Garfinkel, L. (1990) Alcohol drinking and mortality among men enrolled in an American Cancer Society prospective study, *Epidemiology* 1: 342–8.

Breslow, N.E. and Day, N.E. (1980) *Statistical Methods in Cancer Research, Vol. 1*, Lyon: International Agency for Cancer Research.

Dyer, A.R., Stamler, J., Paul, O., Lepper, M., Shekelle, R.B., Mckean, H. and Garside, D. (1980) Alcohol consumption and seventeen-year mortality in the Chicago Western Electric Company Study, *Preventive Medicine* 9: 78–90.

Goddard, E. and Ikin, C. (1988) *Drinking in England and Wales in 1987*, London: HMSO.

Gordon, T. and Kannel, W.B. (1984) Drinking and mortality: the Framingham study, *American Journal of Epidemiology* 120: 97–107.

Humphris, T., Bennett, M. and Ray, C. (1991) *Alcohol Can Damage Your Health*, London: Alcohol Concern.

Klatsky, A.L., Friedman, G.D. and Siegelaub, A.B. (1981) Alcohol and Mortality – a ten-year Kaiser-Permanente experience, *Annals of Internal Medicine* 95: 139–45.

Marmot, M.G., Rose, G., Shipley, M.J. and Thomas, B.J. (1981) Alcohol and Mortality: a U-shaped curve, *Lancet* 14 March: 580–4.

McDonnell, R. and Maynard, A. (1985) Estimation of life-years lost from alcohol-related premature death, *Alcohol and Alcoholism* 20: 435–43.

Payne, C.D., ed. (1985) *The GLIM System Release 3.77 – Manual* Oxford: NAg Ltd.

Petersson, B., Krantz, P., Kristensson, H., Trell, E., and Sternby, N.H. (1984) Alcohol-related death: a major contributor to mortality in urban middle-aged men, *Lancet* 13 November: 1088–90.

Room, R. and Day, N. (1974) Alcohol and mortality, in *Alcohol and Health: New Knowledge*, Washington: USGPO.

Rothman, K.J. (1980) The proportion of cancer attributable to alcohol consumption, *Preventive Medicine* 9: 174–9.

Royal College of General Practitioners (1986) *Alcohol: a Balanced View*, London: RCGP.

Royal College of Physicians (1987) *A Great and Growing Evil*, London: Tavistock.

Schmidt, W. and de Lint, J. (1970) Estimating the prevalence of alcoholism from alcohol consumption and mortality data. *Quarterly Journal of Studies on Alcohol* 31: 957–64.

Shaper, A.G., Wannamethee, G. and Walker, M. (1988) Alcohol and mortality in British men: explaining the U-shaped curve, *Lancet* December 3: 1267–73.

Wilson, P. (1980) *Drinking in England and Wales*, London: HMSO.

4 Alcohol Consumption and Liver Cirrhosis

Although the connection between alcohol consumption and liver damage was noted as long ago as the eighteenth century (Jolliffe and Jellinek, 1941), there was little epidemiological research in this area until the 1970s, stimulated by developing interest in social and medical problems of alcohol consumption.

During the immediate post-war period, various aetiological explanations were advanced in which the association between cirrhosis and alcohol consumption arose from nutritional deficiencies associated with heavy drinking, rather than a hepato-toxic effect of alcohol. While nutritional factors may indeed be associated with both alcohol consumption and liver damage, consensus opinion now holds that such confounding is not sufficient to account for the relation between alcohol and cirrhosis observed in studies on both animals and humans, and that alcohol *per se* has a toxic effect on the liver (Lieber, 1975).

Nevertheless, alcohol is not the only cause of liver cirrhosis. Viral hepatitis may facilitate the development of cirrhosis by affecting the ability of the liver to regenerate (Ipsen, 1950). A number of chemical and pharmaceutical agents are also known to induce chronic liver disease (see Maddrey, 1983).

4.1 The magnitude of the problem

Liver cirrhosis is not a major cause of death in England and Wales. Under the category 'Chronic Liver Disease and Cirrhosis', code 571 of the International Classification of Diseases, there were 1,496 male adult deaths (907 under 65 years of age) and 1,213 female adult deaths (660 under 65) in England and Wales in 1987 (OPCS, 1989). These correspond to annual rates per 1,000,000 of 77 and 58 respectively. Although code 571 includes chronic liver disease other than cirrhosis, diagnostic difficulties and the possible association between alcohol and these other conditions makes it prudent to include all deaths under this code in the present analysis.

An estimate of hospital-treated morbidity may be obtained from the Hospital In-Patient Enquiry, the most recent data being for the year 1985. In that year, from a sample of 1 in 10 of all in-patient discharges and deaths, there were 473 males and 415 females classified under code 571. Thus one may estimate the totals of episodes of treatment in hospital for these conditions in England and Wales as 4,730 and 4,150 respectively.

4.2 The contribution of alcohol consumption to morbidity

Alcoholic liver cirrhosis is a subcategory of code 571, and so it would be possible though naive to use this category as the estimate of cirrhosis due to alcohol consumption. In 1987, a total of 690 liver deaths among men and 412 among women were classified as alcohol-related. There are strong reasons to believe that this assignment is not reliable. In fact, recent research suggests that in England and Wales death certification may under-represent all (not just alcoholic) liver cirrhosis mortality, due to the reluctance of certifying physicians to record this condition as the cause of death, although administrative changes in the mid-1980s may be expected to lead to a reduction in under-recording (Carstairs and Kemp, 1987; Kreitman and Duffy, 1989). An additional reason for using the entire classification is that epidemiological research indicates increased risk of liver cirrhosis at fairly low levels of consumption, and it is unlikely that alcohol-related deaths of low consumers would be correctly identified as such.

Of all the possible approaches to estimation of the influence of alcohol consumption on the above figures, the most satisfactory is based on estimation of the attributable risk along the lines of Section 1.9, and the ideal data source for the purpose of estimating the proportion of cirrhosis mortality or morbidity associated with alcohol consumption would be a large follow-up study of a random sample of the population of England and Wales, with full information of the drinking habits of each subject over the period of study until the development of cirrhosis (morbidity) or death from cirrhosis (mortality). Clearly though, such a study would be hopelessly uneconomic. The low death rate from cirrhosis would necessitate a huge sample size for investigation.

In reality, the data sources available are much more modest, those capable of being used for the purpose of estimating attributable risk of morbidity deriving from two studies in France (Pequignot et al., 1974; Pequignot et al., 1978) and one in Scotland (Chick et al., 1986). These are all case-control studies, that is the alcohol consumption of a sample of cases is compared with that of non-cases. Although relative risks cannot be estimated directly from these studies, odds ratios can be, and, since liver cirrhosis is a rare phenomenon, the odds ratio estimates approximate the relative risks (Cornfield, 1951). A further point to note is that the studies all involve liver cirrhosis patients rather than deaths. It is thus relative risks of morbidity rather than mortality which may be estimated, although it will be useful for illustrative purposes to compare the risk estimates for morbidity to those for mortality. Three large-scale studies of mortality will be used for this purpose, the American Cancer Society Study (Boffetta and Garfinkel, 1990), the Framingham Study (Gordon and Kannel, 1984) and the

Table 4.1: Liver cirrhosis morbidity by alcohol consumption level

	P(1974)			P(1978)			C(1986)	
Consumption (units/wk)	RR	E and W popn	Cons	RR	E and W popn	Cons	RR	E and W popn
						Abst	1.00	0.05
0–16	1.00	0.70	0–16	1.00	0.70	<1	0.73	0.17
17–32	0.66	0.15	17–32	2.91	0.15	1–5	0.92	0.21
33–49	0.78	0.09	33–49	5.61	0.09	6–10	0.99	0.14
50+	7.35	0.06	50+	44.54	0.06	11–20	1.30	0.18
						21–50	2.16	0.19
						51+	8.13	0.06
Total cases	144			184			37	

Honolulu Heart Study (Blackwelder et al., 1980). Although the Kaiser-Permanente study (Klatsky et al., 1981) contains a table relating cirrhosis mortality to alcohol consumption, the matched design of the study renders the marginal rates unsuitable for analysis.

Only one of the three morbidity studies (Pequignot, 1974) includes data concerning women, the other two being restricted to males. Further, in order to apply the results from these studies to the population of England and Wales, the proportion of drinkers in each of the categories used in the original studies in the current population is required. The recent survey 'Drinking in England and Wales in 1987' (Goddard and Ikin, 1988) provides relevant information. The French studies report categories based on grams of absolute alcohol equivalent per day, which entails some transformation and interpolation in the tables of Goddard and Ikin (1988). While the French studies were restricted to liver cirrhosis, the Scottish investigation concerned liver disorders in general, and would be expected to include infectious hepatitis and other liver diseases not associated with alcohol consumption. Thus it must be stressed that the results of the following analyses are no more than indications of the possible impact of alcohol on liver cirrhosis morbidity. There are obvious problems of applying relative risks from one country to the population of a different country, particularly those risks relating to the highest category of consumption, which is usually open at the top, and in which the distributions of consumption may be quite different between the countries. Equally, the heterogeneous nature of the liver disorders considered by Chick et al. (1986) may lead to underestimation of the relation between alcohol and cirrhosis.

4.2.1 Males

Table 4.1 shows the relevant information for all three morbidity studies. The categories used are in all cases those reported in the original works,

Table 4.2: Alcohol-related morbidity in England and Wales males in 1985

	P(1974)	P(1978)	C(1986)
Cases attributable to alcohol	1121	3633	1840
Reference class	0–16 units/wk	0–16 units/wk	abstainers

although for simplicity the measurements in grams/day from the French studies have been converted to units per week, setting 1 unit equal to approximately 8.5 grams. The French studies do not separately identify abstainers, as there were very few such among the cases (only 1 in the 1978 study). The Pequignot (1978) study provided age-standardised results, whereas the data from the others do not appear to be adjusted for age. The higher categories in the French studies involve amounts up to 200 units per week, and it is not possible to estimate England and Wales population proportions at such high values of consumption from the Goddard and Ikin data. Thus there are considerably fewer categories represented in Table 4.1 than in the published French sources, and the relative risk estimates for the highest categories have been calculated by combining the cells of the published tables corresponding to high values.

There are a number of striking differences between the studies, both in terms of presentation and results. First of all, the reference class in the French studies was 0–16 units per week, whereas it is possible to use the abstainers as the reference in the Scottish study. In terms of the relative risks, the Pequignot (1974) results are markedly different from Pequignot (1978), increased risk in the former being confined to the 50+ units/week category. Of course, all these studies are based on relatively small numbers of cases, and a degree of variation is to be expected.

If, for each of the three sets of data, we multiply the relative risks in each category by the corresponding population proportions and add, the result is the coefficient by which the rate in the reference category is multiplied by the impact of alcohol in the population (cf. Section 1.9). Thus, for the Pequignot et al. (1974) study applied to the England and Wales population in 1987, we find that population morbidity is 1.31 times morbidity in the reference class. This implies that using these estimates of relative risk produces an attributable risk of 0.31/1.31 or 23.7%. The same calculation for the 1978 study gives an attributable risk of 76.8%, and the Scottish study an attributable risk of 38.9%. These results may be applied to morbidity statistics to give the figures in Table 4.2, the number of cases which might be attributed to alcohol using the relative risks derived from each of the three studies. The data relating to morbidity are for the year 1985, so differences in population consumption between 1985 and 1987 could lead to further inaccuracies. Finally, it must be acknowledged that morbidity statistics will include repeated admissions of some individuals,

Table 4.3: Alcohol and liver cirrhosis risk in women

Consumption (units/wk)	RR	Population proportion	RR × Pop prop
0–16	1.00	0.960	0.960
17–32	2.83	0.022	0.062
33+	32.97	0.018	0.593
Number of cases	83		

and the frequency of admission may itself be associated with alcohol consumption.

4.2.2 Females

As mentioned earlier, there is only one study to consider, that of Pequignot et al. (1974). The results of the study and corresponding population proportions for England and Wales are reproduced as Table 4.3.

The sum of the last column is 1.615, indicating that 0.615/1.615 or 38% of total morbidity may be attributable to alcohol consumption. This figure corresponds to 1,577 cases of the total estimated morbidity of 4,150.

4.3 Mortality

Since liver cirrhosis is not a common cause of death, as is say heart disease, very large-scale prospective studies would be required to identify the relationship between consumption and harm with any degree of precision. As mentioned earlier, a number of US studies are large enough to permit analysis, and their findings in respect of male subjects only are shown in Table 4.4. Of the three, only the Framingham study (Gordon and Kannell, 1984) reported liver cirrhosis mortality among women, with a total of 10 deaths from a study population of over 2,600. Accordingly, no analysis of female mortality will be attempted. All measurements used to establish categories in the original reports have been recalculated as units per week, and the midpoints of the categories entered as the appropriate values of consumption.

Statistical analysis by means of the GLIM computer package (Payne, 1985) proceeded by fitting a logistic linear regression model to the observed frequencies of death, considered as a binomial random variables with numbers at risk as given in Table 4.4. The numbers at risk in the American Cancer Society Study were estimated from the person-years at risk in the published table by dividing by the length of the follow-up period. Alcohol consumption and its square were fitted as variates, and study fitted as a factor with three levels. The results of fitting and values of the estimates in the best-fitting model are given in Table 4.5.

It can be seen that alcohol consumption accounts for most of the

Table 4.4: Liver cirrhosis mortality by alcohol consumption category (males)

Study	Alcohol consumption	Number of deaths	Number at risk
HHS	0	6	3,747
	4	1	1,316
	14	2	1,583
	35	7	1,232
FS	0	1	402
	4	2	668
	11	0	264
	17	2	175
	30	3	344
	50	3	131
	75	3	122
ACSS	0	155	136,734
	3	31	16,700
	10	44	30,332
	20	82	21,304
	30	67	10,105
	40	71	6,532
	50	39	2,989
	70	153	6,709

deviance in the data, but that a quadratic term in consumption improves the fit further. There is no evidence of significant interaction between study and consumption, indicating that all three studies yield similar estimates of the association between consumption and cirrhosis mortality, although it should be noted that the American Cancer Society Study is preponderantly influential in the analysis due to its large number of respondents. The values

Table 4.5: Model deviances and test statistics – liver cirrhosis mortality

Model	Residual Deviance	Degrees of Freedom	Difference	Degrees of Freedom
Null Fit	806.0	18		
Study	796.1	16	9.9	2
+ Alcohol consumption (linear)	33.7	15	762.4	1
+ Alcohol consumption (quadratic)	16.8	14	16.9	1
+ Study by alcohol Interactions	13.9	10	2.9	4

Effect	Estimate	Standard error
Alcohol consumption (linear)	0.06510	0.00549
Alcohol consumption (quadratic)	−0.0003135	0.000075

Table 4.6: Calculation of attributable risk of liver cirrhosis mortality

Alcohol Consumption (units/wk)	Population Proportion	Relative risk
0	0.05	1.000
0.5	0.17	1.033
3	0.21	1.212
8	0.14	1.650
13	0.11	2.211
18	0.07	2.916
23	0.04	3.787
28	0.05	4.840
33	0.03	6.092
38	0.02	7.547
43	0.03	9.204
48	0.02	11.051
65	0.06	18.301

of the coefficients indicate increasing mortality with level of consumption, but the presence of the vary small quadratic term acts to reduce the slope of the risk relationship slightly.

Attributable risk was calculated on the basis of the figures in Table 4.6. Population proportions and corresponding categories were taken from Goddard and Ikin (1988) Table 2.12 for all males. The highest consumption category in this table is of course open-ended, and a consumption value of 65 units per week has been assumed. Corresponding estimates of relative risk were obtained by applying the coefficient estimates from the logistic-linear model to the category midpoints, which offers a reasonable approximation in the absence of more specific distributional information.

The resulting estimate of attributable mortality is 71.27%, which equates to 1,066 male adult deaths (646 under the age of 65). The rate per million in the reference category, zero consumption, may be estimated as 2.2 for all males. A striking feature is that the estimated attributable risk of mortality from these (American) studies is similar to that for morbidity from Pequignot et al. (1978). Nevertheless, it is important to bear in mind that there are many reasons, discussed in Chapter 3, why findings from studies in one particular country may not be appropriate in another. A further point to note is that, as might be expected, this estimate is considerably greater than 690, which is the number of chronic liver disease deaths attributed to alcohol in the published figures of deaths by cause.

4.4 Conclusion

That alcohol consumption plays a causal role in the development of cirrhosis would not now be disputed, even less that drinking alcohol can be a *direct* cause of death among patients already suffering from cirrhosis.

Nevertheless, the figures presented here can take no account of possible confounding by nutritional factors associated with alcohol consumption and cirrhosis. If such confounding exists, then it is likely that all the estimates of attributable mortality are biased upwards.

Thus no apology need be made for the provision of such widely differing estimates of the impact of drinking on cirrhosis in males. The variability of their results indicates the difficulty of drawing definitive conclusions from small epidemiological investigations, and that caution should be exercised in interpreting the figures for females.

References

Chick, J., Duffy, J.C., Lloyd, G.G. and Ritson, B. (1986) Medical admissions in men: the risk among drinkers, *Lancet*: 1380–3.

Cornfield, J. (1951) A method of estimating comparative rates from clinical data: application to cancer of the lung, breast and cervix, *Journal of the National Cancer Institute* 11: 1269–75.

Goddard, E. and Ikin, C. (1988) *Drinking in England and Wales in 1987*, London: HMSO.

Ipsen, J. (1950) An epidemic of infectious hepatitis, predominantly of adults and highly fatal for elderly women, *American Journal of Hygiene* 51: 225–63.

Jolliffe, N. and Jellinek, E.M. (1941) Vitamin deficiencies and liver cirrhosis in alcoholism, Part VII: Cirrhosis of the liver, *Quarterly Journal of Studies on Alcohol* 2: 544–83.

Kemp, I. and Carstairs, V. (1987) The reliability of death certification as a measure of the level of alcohol problems, *Community Medicine* 9: 146–51.

Kreitman, N. and Duffy, J. (1989) Alcoholic and non-alcoholic liver disease in relation to alcohol consumption in Scotland, 1978–84, *British Journal of Addiction* 84: 607–18.

Lieber, C.S. (1975) Alcohol and the liver: transition from metabolic adaptation to tissue injury and cirrhosis, in Khanna, J.M., Israel, Y. and Kalant, H. (eds) *Alcoholic Liver Pathology*, Toronto: Addiction Research Foundation.

Maddrey, W.C. (1983) Drug-induced chronic active hepatitis, in Cohen, S. and Soloway, R.D. (eds) *Chronic Active Liver Disease*, Edinburgh: Churchill-Livingstone.

Office of Population Censuses and Surveys (1989) *Mortality by Cause 1987*, London: HMSO.

Pequignot, G., Chabert, C., Eydoux, H. and Courcoul, M.A. (1974) Augmentation du risque de cirrhose en fonction de la ration d'alcool, *Revue de l'Alcoolisme* 20: 191–202.

Pequignot, G., Tuyns, A.J. and Berta, J.L. (1978) Ascitic cirrhosis in relation to alcohol consumption, *International Journal of Epidemiology* 7: 113–20.

5 Alcohol-Drinking and Mortality from Diseases of Circulation

Mortality due to diseases of the circulatory system includes various forms of heart disease, such as ischaemic heart disease and hypertension, diseases of the arteries and veins, and cerebrovascular disease. This chapter will consider the epidemiological evidence relating alcohol consumption to cardiovascular disease in general, hypertension and stroke.

Cardiovascular mortality has been extensively investigated in large-scale longitudinal (prospective) population studies, usually of middle-aged male subjects, in several countries. These include the United States, for example the Framingham Study (Gordon et al., 1983), Honolulu Heart Study (Blackwelder et al., 1980), Chicago Western Electric Study (Dyer et al., 1980), Kaiser-Permanente Study (Klatsky et al., 1981), Albany Study (Gordon and Doyle, 1987), Puerto Rico Heart Health Program (Kittner et al., 1983), American Cancer Society Study (Boffetta and Garfinkel, 1990), the Health Professionals Follow-up Study (Rimm et al., 1991); the United Kingdom with the British Regional Heart Study (Shaper et al., 1988) and the Whitehall Study (Marmot et al., 1981); New Zealand with the Auckland study (Jackson et al., 1991); and the Yugoslavian cardiovascular disease study (Kozarevic et al., 1982).

Published reports vary in the level of diagnostic detail provided, most adopting an inclusive approach in which all mortality from circulatory disorders is analysed. This definition therefore includes mortality from cerebrovascular disease, in addition to rheumatic and ischaemic heart disease and hypertensive disease.

Unfortunately from the point of view of this review, the role of alcohol in cardiovascular mortality was not a main topic of investigation *ab initio* in most of the studies. For the most part, alcohol consumption has been measured only at a single point in time, and with rather little attention to detail. In some cases, only a very short dietary recall measure was used, e.g. the Whitehall study used a three-day dietary recall, and the Honolulu Heart Study employed a 24-hour dietary recall as a supplement to questions concerning usual quantity and frequency of drinking. More satisfactory measurement would involve some attempt to map out drinking histories of the study members.

In assessing the role of alcohol in cardiovascular mortality, one may start with the clear and well-known causal effect of alcohol in the development of a congestive cardiomyopathy, ICD 425.5. This is however an extremely rare cause of death, as will be seen later, and it is the possible role of alcohol in heart disease in general which is of far more interest from a public health perspective.

Until fairly recently, it would have been possible to point to a consensus among researchers that available evidence indicated a clear protective effect of alcohol consumption in cardiovascular disease (Marmot, 1984). In some reported datasets, the risks for heavy consumers were greater than for moderate drinkers (a U-shaped curve) although often not as great as the risk among non-drinkers. In others, there was a more or less inverse relation between consumption and risk of cardiovascular mortality. This consensus was not however accepted by the medical establishment as represented by editorials in leading medical journals (Kreitman, 1982; Anon., 1987).

The consensus was challenged by Wannamethee and Shaper (1988), who sought to explain the observed patterns of association as due to the difference in risk between non-drinkers and drinkers, which in their view arises from the unusual characteristics of male non-drinkers. In a later paper, Shaper et al. (1988) subdivide respondents in the British Regional Heart Study into those with previous cardiovascular diagnoses at the start of the study and the rest, and show that for those initially healthy the association between alcohol consumption and cardiovascular mortality is no longer inverse, U-shaped or statistically significant. They then explain the extremely strong inverse relation with a slight upturn in risk for the heaviest drinkers among the other, initially ill, respondents in terms of self-selection. Those who are most ill and therefore most at risk drink the least – because they are ill. The upturn in risk among the heaviest drinkers in this group is explained as an effect of their consumption. While the data for the initially ill group are also consistent with a protective effect of drinking among men with cardiovascular diagnoses, they maintain that such an interpretation does not accord with information concerning changes in drinking habits. It should be noted however that the case put forward is not that alcohol increases overall risk of cardiovascular mortality; indeed, as mentioned earlier, the results for the initially healthy men indicate no relation between alcohol consumption and cardiovascular mortality.

The views of Shaper et al. do not represent a new consensus. Many other researchers continue to maintain the protective effect of alcohol, and indeed there are plausible biological mechanisms which would produce such an effect (Moore and Pearson, 1986). Studies of initially healthy subjects have also shown a protective effect of consumption (see, for example, Dyer et al., 1980; Klatsky et al., 1986). The Whitehall study (Marmot et al., 1981) also addressed this question and found evidence of higher mortality in non-drinkers in both the healthy and unhealthy groups. Similar analyses with similar results were undertaken by Boffetta and Garfinkel (1990), Jackson et al. (1991) and Rimm et al. (1991).The position is therefore one

Table 5.1: Relative risks of mortality from cardiovascular disease from two British studies

a) Marmot et al., 1981, adjusted

Published bands grams/day	units/wk	E&W male pop % (3)	RR compared to '0' band (4)
0	0	5	1.00
0.1–9	1–6	41	0.48
10–34	7–27	34	0.71
34+	28+	20	0.43

b) Shaper et al., 1988, unadjusted

Published bands units/wk	E&W male pop % (3)	RR compared to '0' band (4)
0	5	1.00
<1	16	0.76
1–15	47	0.61
16–42	23	0.47
43+	9	0.69

of controversy rather than consensus, with the majority of researchers in this field at the moment probably inclining to the view that alcohol consumption at moderate levels does indeed have a protective effect.

5.1 Relative risks of male cardiovascular mortality from UK studies

It would be possible to produce extensive tables relating relative risk of cardiovascular mortality and alcohol consumption from various countries, some of which would be quite similar, others rather diverse. Since data are available for UK male samples, it seems most appropriate to consider these in detail. Due to the lack of data concerning women, alcohol and cardiovascular disease, attention will also be restricted to males.

The first thing to notice in Table 5.1 is that the risk to drinkers in all categories is less than the risk to non-drinkers. Although the data from Marmot have been adjusted for age, smoking, blood pressure, cholesterol and grade of employment while the Shaper study figures are unadjusted and indicate that risk in the highest consumption band is more than that for moderate consumers, there is little difference between the pattern of risk in the two parts of the table. England and Wales population proportions in each of the drinking categories are included for the purpose of attributable risk calculations to be reported later.

Table 5.2 shows the relative risk of mortality from cardiovascular disease according to level of alcohol consumption when respondents in the British Regional Heart Study were subdivided according to previous diagnosis.

Table 5.2: Relative risks of cardiovascular mortality from Shaper et al. (1988) with the sample subdivided as with and without previous cardiovascular diagnosis

Published bands units/wk	With previous diagnosis	Without previous diagnosis
	RR wrt '0' band	RR wrt '0' band
0	1.00	1.00
<1	0.91	0.97
1–15	0.64	0.93
16–42	0.38	0.90
43+	0.53	1.39

The reduced risk for drinkers is confined to those men with a previous diagnosis, and as mentioned above may be explained on the basis of their illness influencing their drinking habits. There is no significant relation between alcohol consumption and cardiovascular mortality among those without an initial diagnosis.

5.2 Mortality from cardiovascular disease in England and Wales and attributable risk

5.2.1 Alcoholic cardiomyopathy ICD 425.5

In 1987, there were a total of 60 male deaths from this diagnosis, of which 46 were under the age of 65, the corresponding figures for females being 14 and 11. Respectively, these correspond to annual rates per million of the adult population of 3.1, 2.8, 0.6 and 0.7. Hence this is far from being a major cause of death, or an appreciable risk for the general population.

5.2.2 Diseases of circulation ICD 390 to ICD 459

Again in 1987, total deaths in this category were 132,599 males, of whom 29,588 were under 65, and 138,462 females, 11,272 under 65. Corresponding rates per million are 6,870, 1,790, 6,650 and 685.

Table 5.3 shows that cardiovascular mortality accounts for about 40% of deaths under the age of 65 in men, and 25% of such deaths in women under 65. Thus death from these causes is a major component of premature mortality. Naturally the death rates vary with age, but published studies relating alcohol to mortality do not permit detailed analysis by age.

It is likely to be highly contentious to compute attributable risks of mortality due to alcohol consumption because of the controversy mentioned earlier. These will be disputed by various protagonists in the debate, as will the resulting estimates of individual risk. Nevertheless, the figures in Tables 5.1a and 5.1b may be used to estimate the attributable risk due to alcohol consumption relative to non-drinkers, by multiplying the

Table 5.3: Summary of numbers of deaths and death rates, England and Wales, 1987

	Male		Female	
	all ages	<65	all ages	<65
All causes	280,177	72,214	286,817	44,150
Rate per million	14,513	4,365	14,860	2,690
Diseases of circulation	132,599	29,588	138,463	11,272
Rate per million	6,870	1,790	6,650	685
Alcoholic cardiomyopathy	60	46	14	11
Rate per million	3.1	2.8	0.6	0.7

figures in columns headed (3) and (4) together in each row, and adding over all rows.

Table 5.1a gives the sum of products as 57.42 – that is the actual number of deaths from cardiovascular disease is estimated to be only 57.42% of what it would be if the entire population were non-drinkers. For males under 65, this would result in 21,941 extra deaths, the population's male under-65 death rate in the non-drinker class being thus estimated at 3,120 per million. Calculation from Table 5.1b gives the figure of 62.85%, the corresponding number of deaths avoided being 17,490, and the death rate in the non-drinker category estimated as 2,850 per million.

Applying the relative risks from the tables, one may estimate the annual rates for the various consumption levels as shown in Table 5.4.

It would be unwise to be dogmatic about the effects, protective or otherwise of alcohol-drinking on cardiovascular mortality. In particular, the 'lives saved by alcohol' calculated in the last section cannot be taken too seriously, as the work of Shaper introduces clear doubts as to the nature of the apparent inverse (or occasionally U-shaped) relationship between alcohol consumption and cardiovascular mortality. The risk estimates of Table 5.4 are subject to the same criticism.

One or two things are however clear. First, not all studies agree with Shaper's in finding a protective effect only in those already ill. Second, the

Table 5.4: Estimates of death rates from cardiovascular disease per million in consumption categories – England and Wales males under 65

a) Marmot et al., 1981, adjusted		b) Shaper et al., 1988, unadjusted	
Units of alcohol/wk	Rate per million	Units of alcohol/wk	Rate per million
0	3,100	0	2,800
1–6	1,500	<1	2,200
7–27	2,200	1–15	1,700
28+	1,300	16–42	1,300
		43+	2,000

selection hypothesis advanced by Shaper to account for the apparent protection requires further testing. If Shaper's finding that the apparent protective effect is confined to the ill is substantiated, then the selection hypothesis becomes crucial – there is not a great difference in public health terms between a protective factor which protects the ill against mortality and in the healthy is neutral, and one which protects everyone.

5.3 Alcohol and hypertension

A subcategory of cardiovascular mortality which has been linked with alcohol consumption is hypertensive disease. A recent review of population studies (MacMahon, 1987) considered 30 cross-sectional studies, and noted that the majority of these reported small but significant elevation of blood pressure in consumers of around 35 units per week or more. In 40% of studies, non-drinkers had higher blood pressures than moderate consumers. The author concluded that the long-term effects of restriction of alcohol intake as a public health measure to reduce levels of hypertension required further investigation by means of long-term controlled trials, particularly among moderate consumers. In this section, we will concentrate for the most part on evidence from studies published recently and not considered in the above-mentioned review.

It is clear from experimental work that there is a causal effect of alcohol on blood pressure among normotensives (subjects with normal blood pressure) and that on restriction of alcohol intake blood pressure rapidly returns to normal. There is therefore a consensus of medical opinion concerning the pressor (pressure-elevating) effect of alcohol. It is less clear that alcohol-induced hypertension carries the same constellation of risk of cardiovascular disease as so-called essential hypertension (Beevers and Maheswaran, 1988). However, some studies have shown that alcohol consumption is also associated with essential hypertension, although the relative risks involved tend to be low, typically around 1.5.

A consistent finding from recent studies in countries as far apart as Canada (Buck and Donner, 1987), the United States (Friedman et al., 1982; Weissfeld et al., 1988), Germany (Keil et al., 1989) and Wales (Elliott et al., 1987) is that a weekly consumption in excess of about 30 units increases the risk of hypertension (defined usually as diastolic pressure in excess of 90mm Hg) by about 50% in men. Possible confounding factors controlled for in estimating this relationship include smoking, age, obesity and medication.

More detailed information about risk levels is available in some studies. These tend to support the notion of a threshold effect, although it would be premature to attempt to specify a precise numerical value of consumption at which risk for drinkers starts to exceed that of non-drinkers.

In contrast to the other two studies, the French study in Table 5.5 does not show evidence of a possible protective effect of moderate consumption,

Table 5.5: Relative risk of hypertension by alcohol consumption category

United States (Weissfeld et al., 1988)

	Alcohol Consumption (units per week)				
	Abstainers	<6	6–11	12–23	>24
Relative Risk (males)	1.0	0.93	0.98	1.14	1.50
(females)	1.0	0.91	1.13	1.93	4.57

Canada (Buck and Donner, 1987)

	Alcohol Consumption (units per week)			
	Abstainers	<12	12–47	48+
Relative Risk (males)	1.0	0.69	1.08	1.38
(females)	1.0	0.66	0.72	0.91

France (Lang et al., 1987)

	Alcohol Consumption (units per week)			
	<9	9–26	27–53	54+
Relative Risk (males)	1.00	1.23	1.38	1.95
(females)	1.00	1.44	1.74	2.48

and does not support the notion of a threshold effect. A further British study (Bulpitt et al., 1987) of some 4,000 subjects indicated a threshold of about 50 units per week for men.

It is extremely difficult to discuss risks of hypertension-related mortality on the basis of these studies. Firstly, while the category of hypertensive disease appears in the mortality by cause statistics (Office of Population Censuses and Surveys, 1987), hypertension is also a risk factor for cardio-vascular and cerebrovascular mortality, although as pointed out earlier it is not known whether alcohol-related hypertension carries the same risk as hypertension in general. For completeness, however, there were totals of 1,637 male and 2,123 female deaths in the category of hypertensive disease in England and Wales in 1987. Of these, 386 were males under 65 years of age, the corresponding figure for women being 608. Annual rates for the total adult population by sex are therefore 85 per million for men and 102 for women. As no published studies of mortality from this cause in relation to alcohol have been found, there is little justification for estimating risk of mortality for different levels of consumption.

In the case of morbidity, however, such estimation may be attempted. A

Table 5.6: Estimated prevalence of hypertension by alcohol consumption category

	Alcohol Consumption (units per week)				
	Abstainers	1–5	6–11	12–24	>24
Prevalence % (males)	23	21	23	26	35

major caveat is that age, smoking habits and obesity are important factors affecting the incidence of hypertension, and should be taken into account. No studies have been found which provide sufficient detail to do this, and therefore a global estimate is made, which should be treated with some caution as a rough guide rather than a precise figure.

The prevalence of hypertension among British civil servants was estimated by Bulpitt et al. (1987) as around 25% in both sexes. Assuming that the relative risks from the Weissfeld study (1988) may be applied to prevalence in a British male population, appropriate calculations give prevalences by consumption category as shown in Table 5.6.

A similar calculation has not been attempted for women because the available data are extremely disparate in regard to risk assessment.

As indicated previously, there is no basis on which to calculate the specific impact of alcohol-related hypertension on mortality, and accordingly no attempt is made to calculate the numbers of hypertension-related deaths due to alcohol. For hypertension prevalence as usually defined in the available studies, the attributable risks may be calculated quite easily, but it is important to realise their limited interpretability. What these estimate is the proportion of hypertension which would be eliminated if all alcohol consumption in the population was at the level of the reference category. This presupposes that alcohol-drinking is indeed causally associated with hypertension, and ignores possible interactions with other risk factors.

The first attributable risk estimate is based on the clearest and most common finding. That is that men consuming over 30 units of alcohol per week are 1.5 times more likely to be hypertensive than those consuming between 0 and 30 units per week. In the male population of England and Wales, about 17% drink more than 30 units per week. The calculation therefore gives an attributable risk of 7.8%. That is, 7.8% of all cases of hypertension could be avoided if those drinking more than 30 units per week reduced their consumption to match that in the group drinking less than 30 units per week, if the assumptions hold.

More detailed calculations may be performed by taking abstainers as the reference group. From Table 5.5, one finds for men the values 8.8% (USA) and 14.5% (France) and, from the Canadian study, that hypertension would actually be 5% *more* prevalent if all men were to abstain. No calculation has been attempted for women, as the risk estimates are extremely disparate.

5.4 *Alcohol consumption and cerebrovascular disease*

Although the relation between alcohol and cerebrovascular disease has been moderately frequently researched, there are few studies that have given adequate attention to quantifying alcohol consumption and estimating the risk at different levels. There seems to be a consensus medical opinion that alcohol is implicated in both ischaemic and haemorrhagic stroke, but the mechanisms may be different in the two cases. The statistical evidence is only persuasive in the case of haemorrhagic stroke for men at high levels of consumption. For women, few of whom have very high consumption, there is little statistical evidence. At low levels of consumption, there is some evidence that alcohol is associated with lower risk of stroke as compared with zero consumption.

Animal studies show an effect of heavy alcohol on cerebral blood flow, and indicate that even low alcohol concentrations can produce spasms in isolated arteries, while high concentrations will cause ruptures of blood vessels (Altura and Altura, 1984). Alcohol has been shown to affect blood platelet metabolism and function (Haut and Cowan, 1974) and hence coagulability. The effect of alcohol is also likely to be mediated by blood levels of HDL and LDL cholesterol which respectively rise and fall with increasing intake. This may account for the apparent protective effect of low alcohol consumption on non-haemorrhagic strokes. Reduced coagulability is potentially harmful in haemorrhagic stroke, although it could be of benefit in coronary heart disease (Criqui, 1987).

The most important risk factor for stroke is hypertension and, as seen in the previous section, heavy drinking is known to be a risk factor for hypertension. Even when hypertension is controlled for statistically, heavy drinking remains significantly associated with increased risk of haemorrhagic stroke (Donahue et al., 1986); hence other mechanisms are likely to exist. It is noted that strokes among alcoholics seem to be precipitated during the intoxication itself rather than in the withdrawal syndrome (Hillbom, 1987). Biochemical markers of alcohol intake have been studied and one in particular, gamma-glutamyl transferase, has been reported as showing a very high association with stroke (Gill et al., 1988). There is also an association between acute alcohol intake and atrial fibrillation which is an established precursor of thromboembolic stroke (Wolf et al., 1978; Ettinger et al., 1976). Altogether, despite quite a large number of studies, the possible mechanisms linking acute alcohol intake with stroke are not well understood, and this is acknowledged in the literature (Hillbom, 1987).

In any attempt to answer the question of how much risk of stroke is alcohol-related, the role of confounding variables must be considered. For example, smoking is generally thought to be a risk factor for stroke, but, as it is highly associated with drinking, estimates of the risk attributable to drinking will vary depending on whether smoking, is or is not adjusted for.

If one adjusts for smoking, the alcohol-relative risk will attempt to estimate the increased risk for a person consuming at a given level compared with a person consuming no alcohol, assuming both smoke the same amount. At extreme smoking levels, such a comparison could be rather hypothetical, as it is rare for zero alcohol consumption to be combined with high smoking, or high alcohol with non-smoking. It is also quite likely that for individuals a change in drinking behaviour would be accompanied by a change in smoking behaviour, so that any increased or decreased risk could not be assigned uniquely to one or other factor. In the absence of understanding of causal mechanisms, there is no unique statistical estimate of risk attributable to alcohol. If smoking is adjusted for, there is likely to be an underestimation of the true alcohol effect; if it is not adjusted for, overestimation is likely to result.

While some studies have attempted to control for smoking, which is at least no harder to measure than drinking, similar comments apply to other confounding variables which are even harder to measure. For example, it has been suggested that diet and nutrition could be confounders, as could 'lifestyle' − it being known that in many populations heavy drinkers tend to live in areas with poor accommodation. It is extremely difficult to control adequately for such confounders in a case-control study; and even in population-based studies, such control, although feasible in principle, has rarely been attempted, presumably for reasons of cost.

It has also been suggested that there may be a genetic confounding variable, that is, an inherited predisposition to both alcohol use and risk of stroke (Donahue et al., 1986), but no studies to examine this are known.

More important than these speculations is the problem of adjusting for hypertension. Since this is likely to be an intervening variable between alcohol and stroke, adjusting for it will result in an underestimate of the true alcohol effect, rather as with smoking. It has been found (Donahue et al., 1986) that individual reduction in alcohol intake is associated with reduced blood pressure and reduced risk of stroke.

5.5 Stroke mortality and morbidity in England and Wales

The following data taken from mortality statistics for England and Wales 1986 (Office of Population Censuses and Surveys, 1988) summarise the relative importance of cerebrovascular disease as a cause of death.

Cerebrovascular disease (ICD codes 430–8) accounts for approximately 10% of male deaths and 15% of female deaths. The vast majority of these are at older ages. Of male deaths from these causes, 86% are of men aged 65 and over; of corresponding female deaths, 94% are of women aged 65 and over. For ages under 65, as shown in Table 5.7, cerebrovascular disease is still a more important cause of death for women than men, although death rates are of course lower for women under age 65.

Within the ICD classifications 430–8 the age pattern of mortality varies

Table 5.7: Deaths from cerebrovascular disease at ages 15–64; England and Wales, 1986

Age	15–44			45–64		
	CVD deaths	all deaths	CVD/all %	CVD deaths	all deaths	CVD/all %
Males	404	12,046	3.4	3,329	58,007	5.7
Females	346	6,716	5.2	2,428	34,546	7.2

Death rates per million from cerebrovascular disease: England and Wales, 1986

Age	15–44	45–64	65+
Males	36.3	622	7,646
Females	31.7	451	8,840

strikingly. Table 5.8 shows that the majority of these deaths below age 45 are attributed to sub-arachnoid haemorrhage (ICD 430) whereas above age 65 the majority are 'acute but ill-defined cerebrovascular disease' (ICD 436).

Statistics on morbidity are available only from the Hospital In-Patient Enquiry (Office of Population Censuses and Surveys, 1987), which is not an ideal source. For the last available year, 1985, a 10% sample of all hospitalised patients gives population estimates for England only (i.e. excluding Wales, Scotland and Northern Ireland) as shown in Table 5.7.

Clearly, cerebrovascular disease imposes a large burden on the health service, particularly at older ages. Comparison of Table 5.9 with Tables 5.7 and 5.8 indicates that only around 20% of hospital cases aged under 65 are fatal.

5.6 *Quantitative estimates of the relation between alcohol consumption and stroke*

5.6.1 *The Honolulu Heart Study*

The Honolulu Heart Study (Blackwelder et al., 1980; Donahue et al., 1986; Kagan et al., 1981) was a follow-up study of about 8,000 men of Japanese descent, aged 45–64 on entry to the study. Alcohol consumption was

Table 5.8: Deaths from selected ICD as % of all cerebrovascular deaths

	15–44	45–64	65+
Males			
430 Subarachnoid haemorrhage	54	14	2
431–2 Intracerebral and other haemorrhage	29	20	7
436 Acute but ill-defined CVD	7	47	59
Females			
430 Subarachnoid haemorrhage	63	27	2
431–2 Intracerebral and other haemorrhage	22	19	7
436 Acute but ill-defined CVD	5	39	57

Table 5.9: Estimated prevalence of selected cerebrovascular diagnoses, England 1985

Age	15–44	45–64	All ages
Males			
ICD 430	910	1,240	2,550
431	190	580	1,480
436	320	6,930	32,000
Females			
ICD 430	910	1,840	3,960
431	190	530	1,820
436	160	3,310	39,530

estimated on entry to the study by a questionnaire asking for 'usual monthly intake' of beer, wine and liquor, and by a 24-hour diet recall interview. It is not clear how reliable these measures were over the lengthy period of the study. However, diagnosis of stroke was carefully defined. Table 5.10 shows for various consumption levels the relative risks of stroke mortality in the first nine years of follow-up and relative risks of stroke incidence in the first twelve years of follow-up. For haemorrhagic strokes, the association with alcohol is very evident and statistically significant. For thromboembolic strokes it is much less clear, there being some evidence of reduced risk at moderate consumption levels but excess risk at high consumption.

5.6.2 The Birmingham Study

In this retrospective case-control study (Gill et al., 1986; 1988), 230 stroke

Table 5.10: Relative risks of stroke mortality and incidence by alcohol consumption level: Honolulu Heart Study

Relative risks compared to zero consumption Consumption (grams/day)	Haemorrhagic stroke	Thromboembolic stroke
a) 9-year mortality		
1–6	1.0	1.4
7–15	2.5	0.8
16–39	2.1	0.5
40–59	1.8	1.0
60+	4.2	1.4
b) 12-year incidence		
1–14	2.2 (1.1, 4.2)*	1.0 (0.9, 1.5)
15–39	2.9 (1.4, 5.9)	1.3 (0.9, 1.4)
40+	4.7 (2.4, 9.5)	1.3 (0.9, 1.7)

*95% confidence interval

Table 5.11: Relative risks of stroke incidence by alcohol consumption level: Birmingham study

Consumption grams/day	Men			Women		
	No of cases	RR compared with		No of cases	RR compared with	
		hospital controls	community controls		hospital controls	community controls
1–15	21	0.5	0.5	21	1.1	0.4
16–39	37	1.1	1.1	4	0.5	0.4
40+	41	4.2	1.8	0	–	–

patients of both sexes, aged 20–70, were compared first with a set of hospital controls and later with a set of community controls. Alcohol consumption was assessed by questions on quantity and frequency of intake within a general health questionnaire. For 20% of cases who were in coma or very seriously ill on admission, this was impractical and consumption was estimated by interviews with relatives and friends. 'Binge drinking' was also examined. Stroke diagnosis was carefully defined according to WHO criteria, with discrimination between intracranial haemorrhage and cerebral infarct according to a quantitative scoring method. The majority of cases (80%) were cerebral infarct. However, relative risks for separate categories of stroke were not published. The hospital controls were patients admitted for surgical procedures and were matched on age, sex and race with the cases. The community controls were randomly selected from the workforce of a Birmingham factory but were not individually matched with the cases. Relative risks at various consumption levels were calculated, adjusting for smoking, treatment for hypertension and medication, as shown above.

The only relative risk significantly higher than 1 was for men consuming over 40g/day compared with hospital controls. In the comparison of this group with community controls (among whom consumption was higher than hospital controls), the relative risk of 1.8 was not significantly greater than 1 (95% confidence interval 0.8–4.5). There is clearly only rather weak evidence here for an effect of alcohol on risk of stroke, in the direction of higher risk for men at high consumption levels and lower risk for both sexes at low consumption level. The small number of haemorrhagic strokes among the cases and the pooling of these with infarcts may account for the lack of statistical power. It is also possible that adjusting for smoking and hypertension has removed some of the alcohol effect.

5.6.3 The Gothenburg Cohort Study (Lindegard and Hillbom, 1987)

A Swedish population of over 150,000, aged 30–59 in 1970, was followed up for 10 years. This study is of interest as it relates to a general (urban)

Table 5.12: Relative risks of stroke incidence by alcohol consumption: British Regional Heart Study

Consumption grams/day	Relative risks compared with non- or occasional drinkers	
	Adjusted for age	Adjusted for age, systolic BP and smoking
1–25	0.7	1.0
25–50	1.0	0.9
51+	1.8	1.3

population with very little loss to follow-up. The population is served by a single general hospital, making diagnostic information for the large number of cases reasonably comparable, although only hospital ward information was used for this study rather than special clinical examination. Information on levels of alcohol consumption is not given, but associations were studied between alcoholism (ICD 303) and cerebral infarct. Subarachnoid and intracranial haemorrhages were excluded unless accompanied by infarct. An inner-city area comprising some 30% of the defined population was selected for more intensive study; in this sub-population, there were 536 alcoholism cases and 339 cases of brain infarct. There was significant evidence of a higher risk of infarct among alcoholics, with ratios of observed to expected cases ranging from 4.5 at age 30–49 to 6.0 at age 50–59. However, these estimates are based on small numbers of cases and were for a specifically selected inner-city area. It is not clear to what extent they can be generalised. Within this district, alcoholics accounted for about 7% of cases of infarct or haemorrhage. In a very crude sense, this might be taken as a measure of the contribution of highly excessive drinking to cerebrovascular disease incidence in this population.

5.6.4 The British Regional Heart Study (Shaper et al., 1981; 1991)

This was an eight-year follow-up study of nearly 8,000 men, aged 40–59 in 1978–80, randomly selected from 24 British towns. Alcohol consumption was estimated by questionnaire on entry to the study and classified in four categories. During the follow-up period, 110 men had at least one stroke and 24 of these died within 28 days of the onset of stroke. No analysis of the relation of alcohol to stroke mortality has been published from this study, but relative risks for stroke incidence (ICD 430–8) were calculated as shown in Table 5.12.

Only the age-adjusted relative risk for the heaviest drinkers in Table 5.12 is significantly greater than 1.0. When adjusted for smoking, this risk fell to 1.5, and, after further adjustment for systolic blood pressure to 1.3, only slightly and not significantly in excess of unity. Further analysis divided respondents into those with and without recall of doctor-diagnosed

Table 5.13: Odds ratios of acute
ischaemic stroke: Chicago study

Consumption grams/day	Odds ratio
1–14	1.95
15–39	1.95
40+	2.31

ischaemic heart disease or hypertension at the time of entry to the study. Among the 83% of men with no such previous diagnosis, the relative risk of stroke was 3.8 in the highest consumption category, falling to about 2.0 (but still significantly different from 1.0) after adjustment for age, smoking and systolic blood pressure. By contrast, among those with recall of a previous diagnosis, the relative risk for the heaviest drinkers was less than 1.0. This effect was attributed by the authors to a change in individuals' consumption behaviour following the previous diagnosis (Shaper et al., 1988; see also Chapter 3, and Section 2 of this chapter). The relative risk of 2.0 is in quite good agreement with the Birmingham study (see Table 5.11).

In this study, smoking and systolic blood pressure were considered to be the most important factors affecting risk of stroke, with an estimated relative risk of 12.1 for smokers with systolic blood pressure over 160mm Hg as compared with non-smokers with blood pressure under 160. The effect of smoking adjusted for alcohol consumption was not reported.

5.6.5 *The US Nurses Study (Stampfer et al., 1988)*

Nearly 90,000 female nurses in the United States, aged 34–59 in 1980, were followed up for 4 years with only 2% loss to follow-up. There were 66 cases of ischaemic stroke and 22 cases of subarachnoid haemorrhage. At moderate drinking levels (5–14 g/day), there was a significantly reduced risk of ischaemic stroke (relative risk 0.3, 95% confidence interval 0.1–0.7) and significantly increased risk of subarachnoid haemorrhage (relative risk 3.7, 95% confidence interval 1.0–13.8).

5.6.6 *Chicago Case-control study (Gorelick et al., 1989)*

In this study, 205 middle-aged and elderly acute ischaemic stroke patients were matched with 410 outpatient controls on age, sex, race and method of hospital payment. Table 5.13 displays the odds ratios (approximating the relative risks of stroke as compared with zero consumption).

When smoking and hypertension were controlled for these odds ratios were reduced and, although still exceeding 1.5, were on the borderline of statistical significance.

5.6.7 Case-control study of young adults, Illinois (Oleckno, 1988)

This was a study of 54 stroke cases in patients aged 15–40 from four hospitals in Illinois. Subarachnoid haemorrhage (ICD 430) and transient cerebral ischaemia (ICD 435) were excluded from the study. The cases were frequency-matched on age and sex with 864 controls from the community (case : control ratio 1:16). Alcohol consumption as such was not measured, but individuals were defined as drinkers if they consumed one or more drink per week. The effects of smoking and oral contraceptive use on stroke were also considered and the effect of alcohol adjusted for these. The crude odds ratio of 1.8 was little affected by adjustment for age, sex or race but was reduced to 1.5 after adjustment for smoking. Without this adjustment, the 95% confidence limits for the odds ratio were approximately 1.0 to 3.3; thus the effect was just about statistically significant at conventional levels.

Although this study was weak in regard to the measurement of alcohol and the lack of differentiation between different types of stroke, it is notable that there were 29 female stroke cases and an odds ratio of 2.1 for females. This suggests a much higher relative risk for women than indicated in the Birmingham study.

5.6.8 Finnish studies

Consecutive cases of cerebrovascular disease presented to the University Hospital in Helsinki were analysed by the day of the week on which the strokes occurred. Strokes were classified as 'alcohol-related' if the patient had had alcohol in the 24 hours preceding the stroke or if the stroke was considered to have been provoked by alcohol withdrawal. Whereas 'non alcohol-related' strokes were distributed fairly evenly over all days of the week, 'alcohol-related' strokes accumulated particularly at the weekends – when it is known that alcohol consumption among the Finnish population in general increases markedly. This association would seem difficult to explain without a link between alcohol and risk of stroke. In fact, the different types of stroke had specific patterns, with the subarachnoid haemorrhages and brain infarcts tending to occur on Saturdays and Sundays, during the intoxication itself, while cerebral seizures tended to occur on Sundays and Mondays, during withdrawal.

In the study of the series of subarachnoid haemorrhages (Hillbom and Kaste, 1982), alcohol intoxication was defined as consumption of at least 80g of pure alcohol within a few hours. The 22% of intoxicated cases were compared with intoxication rates derived from a general survey of the Finnish population. It was inferred that intoxication gave a relative risk of subarachnoid haemorrhage of between 2 and 3 for men, and between 2 and 13 for women. For heavy drinking (more than 5 drinks per day), the relative risks were estimated as 2 for men and 7 for women.

5.6.9 Estimates of attributable risk

In order to estimate the level of stroke risk in the United Kingdom that is attributable to drinking, it is necessary to use one or more of the widely varying sets of estimates of relative risk given in this section. As pointed out in Chapter 3, a number of assumptions have to be made in applying a set of relative risks for one population, e.g. the men of Japanese descent in Honolulu, to a completely different UK population. Genetic, dietary, lifestyle and environmental differences between the populations could well make the generalisation untenable.

Following the method of estimating attributable risk in Section 1.9, using estimates from the Honolulu Heart study, Table 5.10a for males aged 45–64 gives the attributable risk of dying from haemorrhagic stroke as 38%, with 544 excess deaths in England and Wales in 1986. Using Table 5.10b, the attributable risk of haemorrhagic stroke incidence is 46%, with about 860 excess cases.

These estimates are extremely high, but the large numbers of unverified assumptions required must be stressed. By contrast, if we use Table 5.11, we find a negative attributable risk of stroke (often called a prevented fraction). This implies a protective effect of alcohol, in the sense that the reduced risk in the low consumption group outweighs the increased risk in the highest consumption group.

The British Regional Heart Study estimated a reduced relative risk for light drinkers and virtually no alcohol effect for moderate drinkers. As a result, the estimates of Table 5.12 imply prevented fractions of 29%, adjusting for age alone, and 0.4% adjusting for age, smoking and blood pressure. As with the Birmingham study, this suggests that overall there are fewer strokes than there would be if the whole population were teetotal. Using the estimates from Shaper et al. (1991) for those without previous diagnosis of disease, there is a small attributable risk of 3%. The low estimate of attributable risk from this study may be due in part to inadequate precision in the measurement and classification of alcohol consumption.

The Chicago study of Table 5.13 implies an attributable risk of 47% which agrees remarkably well with the Honolulu study, although they refer to different types of stroke.

To conclude, there is an extensive body of evidence relating alcohol to stroke, although detailed understanding of the mechanisms is lacking. The risk is particularly associated with heavy alcohol consumption, whereas low consumption may actually confer some protection against stroke. Although cerebral infarcts are rare in young people, association between heavy drinking and brain infarct in young adults has been observed in several countries (Hillbom, 1987).

Estimates of relative risk vary widely and depend on sex, level of consumption, type of stroke and whether other important factors are adjusted for. An overall attributable risk of about 40% is supported by three of the studies considered. There is a need for further studies that quantify the level of alcohol more precisely, though it must be recognised that there are severe practical constraints to accomplishing this.

References

Altura, B.M. and Altura, B.T. (1984) Alcohol, the cerebral circulation and strokes, *Alcohol* 1: 325–31.

Anon. (1987) Dying for a drink? *Lancet* ii: 1249–50.

Beevers, D.G. and Maheswaran, R. (1988) Does alcohol cause hypertension or pseudo-hypertension? *Proceedings of the Nutrition Society* 47: 111–14.

Blackwelder, W.C., Yano, K., Rhoads, G.G., Kagan, A., Gordon, T. and Palesch, Y. (1980) Alcohol and mortality: the Honolulu heart study, *American Journal of Medicine*, 68: 164–9.

Boffetta, P. and Garfinkel, L. (1990) Alcohol-drinking and mortality among men enrolled in an American Cancer Society prospective study, *Epidemiology* 1: 342–8.

Buck, C.W. and Donner, A.P. (1987) Factors affecting the incidence of hypertension, *Canadian Medical Association Journal* 136: 357–60.

Bulpitt, C.J., Shipley, M.J. and Semmence, A. (1987) The contribution of a moderate intake of alcohol to the presence of hypertension, *Journal of Hypertension* 5: 85–91.

Criqui, M.H. (1987) The roles of alcohol in cardiovascular disease, *Acta Medica Scandinavica* suppl. 717: 73–85.

Donahue, R.P., Abbott, R.D., Reed, D.M. and Yano, K. (1986) Alcohol and haemorrhagic stroke: the Honolulu Heart Program, *Journal of the American Medical Association* 255: 2311–14.

Dyer, A.R., Stamler, J., Paul, O., Lepper, M., Shekelle, R.B., Mckean, H. and Garside, D. (1980) Alcohol consumption and seventeen-year mortality in the Chicago Western Electric Company Study, *Preventive Medicine* 9: 78–90.

Elliott, P., Fehily, A.M., Sweetnam, P.M. and Yannell, J.W. (1987) Diet, alcohol, body mass and social factors in relation to blood pressure: the Caerphilly Heart Study, *Journal of Epidemiology and Community Health* 41: 37–43.

Ettinger, P.O., Wu, C.F., De La Cruz, C.Jr., Weisse, A.B., Ahmed, S.S. and Regan, T.J. (1978) Arrhythmia and the 'holiday heart': alcohol-associated cardiac rhythm disorders, *American Heart Journal* 95: 555–562.

Friedman, G.D., Klatsky A.L. and Siegelaub, A.B. (1982) Alcohol, tobacco and hypertension, Hypertension 4: suppl. III, 143–50.

Gill, J.S., Shipley, M.J., Hornby, R.H., Gill, S.K. and Beevers, D.G. (1988) A community case-control study of alcohol consumption in stroke, *International Journal of Epidemiology* 17: 542–7.

Gill, J.S., Zezulka, A.V., Shipley, M.J., Gill, S.K. and Beevers, D.G. (1986) Stroke and alcohol consumption, *New England Journal of Medicine* 315: 1041–6.

Goddard, E. and Ikin, C. (1988) *Drinking in England and Wales in 1987*, London: HMSO.

Gordon, T. and Doyle, J.T. (1987) Drinking and mortality: the Albany study, *American Journal of Epidemiology* 125: 263–70.

Gordon, T. and Kannell, W.B. (1983) Drinking habits and cardiovascular disease: the Framingham study, *American Heart Journal* 105: 667–73.

Gorelick, P.B., Rodin, M.B., Langenberg, P., Hier, D.B. and Costigan, J. (1989) Weekly alcohol consumption, cigarette smoking and the risk of ischaemic stroke: results of a case-control study at three urban medical centres in Chicago, Illinois, *Neurology* 39: 339–43.

Haut, M.J. and Cowan, D.H. (1974) The effect of ethanol on hemostatic properties of human blood platelets, *American Journal of Medicine* 56: 22–3.

Hillbom, M.E. (1987) What supports the role of alcohol as a risk factor for stroke? *Acta Medica Scandinavica* suppl. 717: 93–106.

Hillbom, M. and Kaste, M.D. (1982) Alcohol intoxication: a risk factor for primary subarachnoid hemorrhage, *Neurology* 32: 706–11.

Jackson, R., Scragg, R. and Beaglehole, R. (1991) Alcohol consumption and risk of coronary heart disease, *British Medical Journal* 303: 211–16.

Keil, U., Chambless, L. and Remmers, A. (1989) Alcohol and blood pressure – results from the Lübeck Blood Pressure Study, *Preventive Medicine* 18: 1–10.

Kittner, S.J., Garcia-Palmieri, M.R., Costas, R., Cruz-Vidal, M., Abbott, R.D. and Havelik, J. (1983) Alcohol and coronary heart disease in Puerto Rico, *American Journal of Epidemiology* 117: 538–50.

Klatsky, A.L., Friedman, G.D., Siegelaub, A.B. and Gerard, M.J. (1977) Alcohol consumption and blood pressure: Kaiser-Permanente Multiphasic Health Examination data, *New England Journal of Medicine* 296: 1194–200.

Klatsky, A.L., Friedman, G.D. and Siegelaub, A.B. (1981) Alcohol and Mortality – a ten-year Kaiser-Permanente experience, *Annals of Internal Medicine* 95: 139–45.

Klatsky, A.L., Armstrong, M.A. and Friedman, G.D. (1986) Relations of alcoholic beverage use to subsequent coronary artery disease hospitalisation, *American Journal of Cardiology* 58: 710–14.

Kozarevic, D., Demirovic, J., Gordon, T., Kaelber, C.T., McGee, D. and Zukel, W.J. (1982) Drinking habits and coronary heart disease: the Yugoslavia cardiovascular disease study, *American Journal of Epidemiology* 116: 748–58.

Kreitman, N. (1982) The perils of abstention, *British Medical Journal* 284: 444–5.

Lang, T., Degoulet, P., Aime, F., Devries, C., Fouriaud, C. and Jacquinet-Salord, M.C. (1987) Relationship between alcohol consumption and hypertension prevalence and control in a French population, *Journal of Chronic Diseases* 40: 713–20.

Lindegard, B. and Hillbom, M. (1987) Associations between brain infarction, diabetes and alcoholism: observations from the Gothenburg cohort study, *Acta Neurologica Scandinavica* 75: 195–200.

MacMahon, S. (1987) Alcohol consumption and hypertension, *Hypertension* 9: 111–21.

Marmot, M.G., Rose, G., Shipley, M.J. and Thomas, B.J. (1981) Alcohol and Mortality: a U-shaped curve, *Lancet* 14 March: 580–4.

Marmot, M.G. (1984) Alcohol and coronary heart disease, *International Journal of Epidemiology* 13: 160–7.

Moore, R.D. and Pearson, T. (1986) Moderate alcohol consumption and coronary heart disease: a review, *Medicine* 65: 242–67.

Office of Population Censuses and Surveys (1987) *Hospital In-patient Enquiry 1985*, London: HMSO.

Office of Population Censuses and Surveys (1988) *Mortality Statistics – Cause 1986*, London: HMSO.

Office of Population Censuses and Surveys (1989) *Mortality Statistics – Cause 1987*, London: HMSO.

Oleckno, W.A. (1988) The risk of stroke in young adults: an analysis of the contribution of cigarette smoking and alcohol consumption, *Public Health* 102: 45–55.

Rimm, E.B., Giovanucci, E.L., Willett, W.C., Colditz, G.A., Ascherio, A., Rosner, B. and Stampfer, M. (1991) Prospective study of alcohol consumption and risk of coronary disease in men, *Lancet*, 338: 464–8.

Shaper A.G., Pocock, S.J., Walker, M., Cohen, N.M., Wale, C.J. and Thomson A.G. (1981) British Regional Heart Study: cardiovascular risk factors in middle-aged men in 24 towns, *British Medical Journal* 283: 179–86.

Shaper, A.G., Wannamethee, G. and Walker, M. (1988) Alcohol and mortality in British men: explaining the U-shaped curve, *Lancet* December 3: 1267–73.

Shaper, A.G., Phillips, A.N., Pocock, S.J., Walker, M. and Macfarlane, P.W. (1991) Risk factors for stroke in middle-aged British men, *British Medical Journal* 302: 1111–15.

Stampfer, M.J., Colditz, G.A., Willett, W.C., Speizer, F.E. and Hennekens, C.H. (1988) A prospective study of moderate alcohol consumption and the risk of coronary disease and stroke in women, *New England Journal of Medicine* 319: 267–73.

Wannamethee, G. and Shaper, A.G. (1988) Men who do not drink: a report from the British Regional Heart Study, *International Journal of Epidemiology* 17: 307–16.

Weissfeld, J.L., Johnson, E.H., Brock, B.M. and Hawthorne, V.M. (1988) Sex and age interactions in the association between alcohol and blood pressure, *American Journal of Epidemiology* 128: 559–69.

Wolf, P.A., Dawber, T.R. and Thomas, H.E. (1978) Epidemiologic assessment of chronic atrial fibrillation and the risk of stroke: the Framingham study, *Neurology* 28: 973–7.

6 Alcohol and Cancer Risk

There is considerable evidence for the carcinogenicity of alcohol in humans. The International Agency for Research on Cancer presented the findings of an expert working group in a monograph (1988), including site-specific reviews and informally summarising a substantial body of material. The conclusion is that alcohol is causally related to cancers of the oral cavity, pharynx, larynx, oesophagus and liver.

The IARC monograph is an invaluable bibliographic and archival source. This chapter is intended to complement its epidemiological content by updating the material reviewed on cancers of the mouth, pharynx, larynx, oesophagus, stomach, colon, rectum, pancreas, liver, lung, breast and bladder, and performing a more quantitative summary in so far as this is possible. For each site, answers to the following questions are sought:

1. What is the quality and quantity of research on the subject?
2. If the available studies, or a subset thereof, can be combined in a quantitative overview, what is the overall effect of alcohol drinking on risk, adjusting for potential confounding variables such as smoking?
3. Is there a consensus on a biological mechanism of effect on risk?
4. What proportion of cases of the disease can be attributed to alcohol drinking?

Quantitative overview was performed using Woolf's (1955) method, after logistic regression analysis (Breslow and Day, 1980), taking weighted averages of the log odds ratio for drinkers relative to non-drinkers or the trend in log-odds ratio with amount of alcohol consumed. For the latter, alcohol consumption was expressed as litres of ethanol per week, using midpoints of quoted categories and converting numbers of beverages to ethanol equivalents where necessary. Calculation of attributable risk is described in Chapter 1.

6.1 Alcohol and oropharyngeal cancer

Here we review all major studies of alcohol consumption and oral and pharyngeal cancer risk (including hypopharynx). Studies assessing risk of cancers of the above sites combined with oesophagus and larynx as one overall site were excluded.

6.1.1 Published research

Table 6.1 shows the studies reviewed which assess alcohol consumption and oral cancer risk. Fifteen studies were reviewed. Of these, thirteen were case-control studies and two were cohort studies following up alcoholics. Of the case-control studies, all but one (Hirayama, 1966) found significant or suggestive increases in risk to be associated with high alcohol consumption. Eight (Martinez, 1969; Bross and Coombs, 1976; Graham et al., 1977; Williams and Horm, 1977; Brugere et al., 1986; Notani, 1988; Franco et al., 1989; Sankaranarayanan et al., 1989b) of the case-control studies reported a significant or suggestive increase in risk after adjustment for smoking or chewing habits. Both of the cohort studies reported significantly increased risks associated with alcoholism.

Thirteen studies of pharyngeal cancer were reviewed (see Table 6.2 for details). Nine were case-control studies, and four were cohort studies following up alcoholics. Of the case-control studies, all reported a significant or suggestive increase in risk with high consumption. For six of these (Martinez, 1969; Williams and Horm, 1977; Olsen et al., 1985; Brugere et al., 1986; Notani, 1988; Tuyns et al., 1988), the effect was adjusted for smoking or chewing habits. All cohort studies found a significant increase in risk among alcoholics.

Table 6.3 shows those studies assessing the effect of alcohol on oral and pharyngeal cancers as a single site. There were seven such studies, three case-control, three cohort studies following up alcoholics and one cohort study of brewery workers. The three case-control studies found significant increases in risk in association with high consumption, adjusting for smoking. One (Blot et al., 1988) found an interaction between smoking and drinking such that the risk associated with both habits simultaneously was higher than that expected from combination of the separate risk estimates for the two habits. All the studies of alcoholics found significantly increased risks in association with alcoholism. No significantly increased risk was noted among brewery workers (Jensen, 1979).

The overall impression of the above is that alcohol does have a predisposing effect to both oral and pharyngeal cancers, and that this effect is not entirely attributable to tobacco habits. There were no direct prospective studies of alcohol consumption *per se* and risk, but the results from the case-control studies are fairly clear.

6.1.2 Partial quantitative overview

Alcohol as a binary risk factor. Table 6.4 shows relative risks of oral cancer for drinkers compared to non-drinkers, in those studies reporting the information, with the combined estimate using Woolf's (1955) method. Overall, the combined estimate of 2.17 is reduced to 1.40 when attention is restricted to those studies giving sufficient information to obtain a

Table 6.1: Studies of cancer of the oral cavity reviewed

Study	Design and methods	Summary of results
Wynder et al., 1957	Case-control, 462 cases, 207 controls (all male). Five daily consumption categories.	Increasing risk with increasing consumption (RR = 5.2 for > 6 drinks/day vs none).
Vincent and Marchetta, 1963*	Case-control. 42 cases, 150 controls. Three daily consumption categories.	Increasing risk with increasing consumption (RR = 9.7 for >2 oz/ day).
Hirayama, 1966*	Case-control. 76 cases, 228 controls. Drinkers vs non-drinkers.	No significant effect adjusted for chewing tobacco or betel (Sri Lankan study).
Sundby, 1967*	Cohort. 1,963 alcoholics followed up for mortality.	Significantly increased risk for alcoholics (RR = 5.0).
Martinez, 1969	Case-control. 138 cases, 138 controls matched for age, sex and smoking. Four daily consumption categories.	Increased risk with increased consumption (RR = 2.5 for 5+ drinks/day vs none).
Bross and Coombs, 1976	Case-control. 145 female cases, 1,973 hospital controls. Three monthly consumption categories.	Significantly increased risk with high consumption among smokers (RR = 3.4 for heavy drinking vs none).
Graham et al., 1977	Case-control. 584 male cases, 1,222 hospital controls. Four weekly consumption categories.	Significantly increased risk with high consumption (RR = 1.7 for 7+ drinks/day) adjusted for smoking.
Williams and Horm, 1977	Case-control. 190 cases, 5,566 controls. Lifetime consumption in three categories.	Significant increase in risk with high consumption, adjusted for tobacco smoking.
Elwood et al., 1984	Case-control. 133 cases, 133 hospital controls. Five weekly consumption categories.	Significant increase in risk with high consumption unadjusted. Smoking-adjusted analyses for combined oral, pharynx and larynx cancers shows significant effect of alcohol.
Bruyere et al., 1986	Case-control. 856 male cases of oral cavity cancer, approx. 2,000 hospital controls. Four daily consumption categories.	Significant increase in risk with high consumption excluding 97 lip cancer cases (RR = 70.3 for 160g/day vs 0–39 g/ day) adjusted for smoking.

Table 6.1: (*Continued*)

Study	Design and methods	Summary of results
Notani, 1988	Case-control. 217 male cases, 162 hospital controls. Drinkers vs non-drinkers.	Significant increase in risk with drinking but reported results difficult to interpret due to possible interaction with age.
Prior, 1988	Cohort. 876 male alcoholics followed up for incidence.	Significant increase in risk with alcoholism (RR = 9.1).
Franco et al., 1989	Case-control. 232 cases, 464 hospital controls. Lifetime consumption in six categories.	Significant increase in risk with high consumption (RR = 8.5 for highest vs lowest) adjusted for smoking.
Sankaranarayanan et al., 1989a	Case-control. 228 cases, 453 hospital controls matched for age, sex and religion. Three drinking categories.	Significant increase in risk associated with drinking, losing its significance when adjusted for tobacco smoking and tobacco/betel chewing.
Sankaranarayanan et al., 1989b	Case-control. 187 cases, 895 hospital controls. Drinkers vs non-drinkers.	Significant increase in risk associated with drinking adjusted for tobacco (RR = 1.9) and betel/ tobacco chewing.

*Publication not available, results obtained from IARC monograph.

tobacco-adjusted estimate. Although the latter's significance is borderline, it is likely that the effect is a real one but that the three studies alone do not have sufficient power to show the result as significant.

For pharyngeal cancer (Table 6.5), a combined estimate of 2.83 was obtained, although in the one study with adjustment for smoking (Martinez, 1969) the estimate was 1.49. Again it is likely that the effect is present but we have not the power to detect it. This is a symptom of restriction to those studies reporting the data in such a way as to be able to combine the results with other studies.

Dose-response. Dose response was measured by trends in the log-odds ratio relative risk estimated with increasing consumption in ml/day of ethanol. For those studies reporting consumption in quantitative categories, the midpoint of each category was taken as the estimated median consumption for that category, and expressed in ml/day of ethanol. Trends were estimated by logistic regression and combined by Woolf's (1955) method.

Results for oral cavity cancers are shown in Table 6.6. The combined estimate of risk is equivalent to a 35% increase in risk with an increased

Table 6.2: Studies of alcohol and pharyngeal cancer reviewed

Study	Design and methods	Summary of results
Wynder et al., 1957	Case-control. 81 male cases, 207 controls. Five daily consumption categories.	Increased risk with high consumption (RR = 7.7 for >6 drinks/day vs non-drinkers).
Vincent and Marchetta, 1963*	Case-control. 40 cases, 150 controls. Three daily consumption categories.	Increased risk with high consumption (RR from 52.5 to 82.0 depending on site).
Sundby, 1967*	Cohort. 1,693 male alcoholics followed up for mortality.	Significant increase in risk with alcoholism (RR = 4.4).
Martinez, 1969	Case-control. 45 cases, 45 age, sex and tobacco matched controls. Four daily consumption categories.	Significant increase in risk associated with high consumption (RR = 5.8 for 5+ drinks/day vs none).
Hakulinen et al., 1974	Cohort. Approx. 210,000 alcoholics and alcohol abusers followed up for incidence.	Significant increase in risk with chronic alcoholism.
Adelstein and White, 1976	Cohort. 2,070 alcoholics followed up for mortality.	Significant increase in risk (RR = 6.7) associated with alcoholism.
Williams and Horm, 1977	Case-control. 73 cases, 5,566 controls. Lifetime exposure in three categories.	Significant increase in risk with high consumption (RR = 6.2 for males, 17.0 for females for highest vs lowest) adjusted for smoking.
Elwood et al., 1984	Case-control. 87 cases, 87 hospital controls. Five consumption categories.	Significant increase in risk with high consumption (RR = 4.5 for highest vs lowest).
Olsen et al., 1985	Case-control. 32 cases of hypopharyngeal cancer, 1,141 controls. Two categories of weekly consumption.	Non-significant increase in risk with high consumption (RR = 1.8), adjusted for smoking.
Bruyere et al., 1986	Case-control. 1,000 male cases, approx. 2,000 controls. Four daily consumption categories.	Significant increase in risk with consumption (RR = 70.3 for oropharynx, 134.1 for hypopharynx for lowest vs highest).
Notani, 1988	Case-control. 166 cases, 162 hospital controls. Drinkers vs non-drinkers.	Significant increase in risk with alcohol use. Possible interaction with age.
Prior, 1988	Cohort. 1,110 alcoholics (876 male) followed up for incidence.	Significant increase in risk with alcoholism (RR = 13.5).
Tuyns et al., 1988	Case-control. 281 male hypopharynx cases, 3,057 controls. Five daily consumption categories.	Significant increase in risk with high consumption, adjusted for smoking (RR = 12.5 for highest vs lowest categories).

*Publication unavailable, results obtained from IARC monograph

Table 6.3: Studies of oropharyngeal cancer as a single site

Study	Design and Methods	Summary of results
Keller and Terris, 1965*	Case-control. 134 male cases, 134 controls. Four daily consumption categories. Matched for smoking.	Significant increase in risk associated with high consumption (RR = 3.7 for >38g/day vs none).
Feldman et al., 1975*	Case-control. 96 male cases, 182 controls. Four daily consumption categories.	Significant increase in risk with high consumption, adjusted for tobacco (RR = 4.5 for >140g/day vs none).
Monson and Lyon, 1975	Cohort. 1382 alcoholics followed up for mortality.	Significant increase in risk with alcoholism (RR = 3.3).
Jensen, 1979	Cohort. 14313 male brewery workers followed up for incidence.	No significant difference between brewery workers and population.
Robinette et al., 1979	Cohort. 4401 male alcoholics and 4401 controls followed up for mortality.	Significant increase in risk in alcoholics (RR = 2.2).
Schmidt and Popham, 1981	Cohort. 9,889 male alcoholics followed up for mortality.	Significant increase in risk with alcoholism (RR = 4.2).
Blot et al., 1988	Case-control. 1,114 cases, 1,268 controls. Five weekly consumption categories.	Significant increase in risk with high consumption (RR = 8.8 for highest vs lowest in men and 9.1 in women). Synergistic interaction with smoking in men.

*Publication unavailable, results obtained from IARC monograph.

consumption of one pint of beer per day. Restricting attention to the two studies yielding smoking-adjusted trends, the combined estimate is equivalent to an increase in risk of 19% for an increased consumption of one pint of beer daily. In both cases, there is significant heterogeneity among studies, but all studies have positive trends.

Results for pharyngeal cancer are shown in Table 6.7. The combined estimate is equivalent to an increased risk of 1.41 with an increased consumption of one pint of beer per day. Again, there is significant heterogeneity among studies but the trends are all positive. In the one study providing a smoking-adjusted trend (Martinez, 1969), the estimate is 0.0103, equivalent to a 24% increase in risk with an increased daily consumption of one pint of beer.

6.1.3 Is there a biological relationship?

The results above suggest that there is an effect of alcohol not entirely

Table 6.4: Relative risks for drinkers compared to non-drinkers for cancers of the oral cavity

Study	Adjusted for tobacco	RR	95% CI	Significance
Wynder et al., 1957	No	1.97	(0.90, 4.33)	ns
Martinez, 1969	Yes	1.11	(0.65, 1.86)	ns
Bross and Coombs, 1976	Yes	1.48	(0.87, 2.49)	ns
Williams and Horm, 1977	No	2.66	(2.01, 3.52)	p<0.001
Notani, 1988	No	1.67	(1.07, 2.59)	p<0.05
Sankaranarayanan et al., 1989a	No	3.19	(2.03, 5.02)	p<0.001
Sankaranarayanan et al., 1989b	Yes	1.87	(1.03, 3.45)	p<0.05
All studies		2.17	(1.82, 2.58)	p<0.001

Significant heterogeneity among studies p<0.01

Studies adjusted for smoking		1.40	(0.96, 2.02)	0.1>p>0.05

No significant heterogeneity among studies

attributable to co-carcinogenesis with other substances. Alcohol may predispose to oral cancer by direct damage to mucosal tissue, by depressing immunity or by compromising nutritional status. Other possible indirect or co-carcinogenic effects could be irritation of tissue which causes increased susceptibility to other carcinogens, or alcohol acting as a solvent for tobacco carcinogens (Smith, 1982; Blot et al., 1988). The IARC monograph (1988) concludes that alcohol is causally related to oral cancer. This is reasonable since its effect cannot be consistently annulled by adjustment for other known factors. Nevertheless, it is not known by what mechanism the carcinogenic effect works. It is likely to be a combination of the above paths.

6.1.4 Attributable risks

Calculations of attributable risks, and hence the potential deaths avoided by altering drinking habits, can be made using deaths from the disease in question and prevalence of the risk factors in the population. In England and Wales in 1987, there were 589 deaths among males and 377 among females

Table 6.5: Relative risks for drinkers compared to non-drinkers for pharyngeal cancer

Study	Adjusted for tobacco	RR	95% CI	Significance
Martinez, 1969	Yes	1.49	(0.53, 4.14)	ns
Williams and Horm, 1977	No	3.49	(2.15, 5.65)	p<0.001
Notani, 1988	No	2.66	(1.71, 4.13)	p<0.001
All studies		2.83	(2.07, 3.86)	p<0.001

No significant heterogeneity among studies

Table 6.6: Trends in the log-odds ratio with increasing alcohol consumption in ml/day, for cancer of the oral cavity

Study	Adjusted for tobacco	Trend	SE	Significance
Wynder et al., 1957	No	0.0155	0.0024	p<0.001
Martinez, 1969	Yes	0.0073	0.0023	p<0.001
Bross and Coombs, 1976	Yes	0.0575	0.0165	p<0.001
Graham et al., 1977	No	0.0267	0.0041	p<0.001
Elwood et al., 1984	No	0.0183	0.0048	p<0.001
All studies		0.0142	0.0014	p<0.001
Significant heterogeneity among studies p<0.001				
Studies adjusted for smoking		0.0083	0.0023	p<0.001
Significant heterogeneity between studies p<0.001				

from oral cancer, excluding oropharynx, nasopharynx, hypopharynx and salivary glands (OPCS 1989). Prevalence of drinkers (at all) in England and Wales is estimated as 95% for males and 92% for females (Goddard and Ikin, 1989). In combination with the combined estimate of relative risk in Table 6.4, unadjusted for tobacco habits, we have attributable risks of 53% in males and 52% in females, yielding a potential number of deaths avoided by eliminating *all* drinking of 508 per year in England and Wales. If we use the tobacco-adjusted relative risk of 1.40, we obtain attributable risks of 28% in men and 27% in women, and a total of 267 deaths avoided. The latter figure is probably closer to the truth.

The above are the deaths avoided by eliminating all drinking. If we aim instead to reduce average consumption, we can estimate the potential numbers of deaths avoided using the trend estimates in Table 6.6. The median consumption in England and Wales can be estimated from the data in Goddard and Ikin (1989) as 21ml/day in men and 5ml/day in women. Using the combined trend estimate of 0.0142, unadjusted for smoking, halving the above consumption figure would lead to risk reductions of 14%

Table 6.7: Trends in the log odds ratio relative risk of pharyngeal cancer with increasing alcohol consumption in ml/day

Study	Adjusted for tobacco	Trend	SE	Significance
Martinez, 1969	Yes	0.0103	0.0037	p<0.01
Elwood et al., 1984	No	0.0281	0.0055	p<0.001
Olsen et al., 1985	No	0.0321	0.0143	p<0.05
All studies		0.0166	0.0030	p<0.001

Significant heterogeneity among studies p<0.001

in men and 3% in women, yielding a total number of deaths avoided of 94. The corresponding results using the smoking-adjusted estimate, 0.0083, are risk reductions of 8% in men and 2% in women, with a total saving of 55 deaths per year.

With respect to pharyngeal cancer, there were 238 deaths in men and 172 in women in England and Wales in 1987 (OPCS), excluding naso-pharynx but including hypopharynx. The combined relative risk estimate for any drinking is given as 2.83 in Table 6.6. Together with the prevalence of 95% and 92% in men and women, this yields an attributable risk of 63% in both men and women, and a potential avoidance of 258 deaths per year. The tobacco-adjusted relative risk of 1.49 yields attributable risks of 32% in men and 31% in women, giving a potential 129 lives saved by elimin-ating *all* drinking. The true figure is likely to lie between the two. Although the smoking-adjusted figure would normally be preferable, it is based on a small number of cases (45) and hence is not reliable.

Using the median estimates of consumption above, and postulating cutting these by half again, the combined unadjusted trend estimate of 0.0116 from Table 6.7 confers reductions in risk of 16% in men and 4% in women, yielding a total potential saving of 45 deaths per year in England and Wales. Using the tobacco-adjusted estimate of 0.0103, the correspond-ing figures are risk reductions of 10% in men and 3% in women, and a total number of deaths avoided of 29. Again, the latter figure should be inter-preted cautiously, as it is based on 45 cases.

6.2 Alcohol and laryngeal cancer

6.2.1 Published research

Twenty-two studies were reviewed and are summarised in Table 6.8. Sixteen studies were of case-control design, one was a cohort study on male brewery workers and the remaining five were cohort studies on alcoholics.

Of the case-control studies, thirteen (Wynder et al., 1956; Vincent and Marchetta, 1963; Spalajkovic, 1976; Wynder et al., 1976; Williams and Horm, 1977; Hinds et al., 1979; Burch et al., 1981; Elwood et al., 1984; Brugere et al., 1986; Zagraniski et al., 1986; De Stefani et al., 1987; Guenel et al., 1988; Tuyns et al., 1988) found significant associations of alcohol with risk, high consumption in all cases being associated with high risk. All but two (Vincent and Marchetta, 1963; Spalajkovic, 1976) were smoking-adjusted results.

Of the cohort studies on alcoholics, three (Sundby, 1967; Monson and Lyon, 1975; Schmidt and Popham, 1981) found significant increases in association with alcoholism. The study of brewery workers (Jensen, 1979) who had higher beer intakes than the general population found that these workers had twice the risk of the rest of the population.

If there can be said to be a gap in the research, it is the absence of direct

Table 6.8: Studies of alcohol consumption and laryngeal cancer

Study	Design and Methods	Summary of qualitative results
Wynder et al., 1956	Case-control. 209 male cases, 209 hospital controls. Beverage-specific analyses.	Increased risk with high consumption, significant when adjusted for smoking.
Vincent and Marchetta, 1963	Case-control. 23 male cases, 100 controls. Two consumption categories (>47g/day, <47g/day)	Significant increase in risk in higher consumption group, compared to 47 g or more, not adjusted for smoking.
Sundby, 1967	Cohort. 1,693 male alcoholics followed up for mortality.	Significantly elevated risk in alcoholics.
Hakulinen et al., 1974	Cohort. Roughly 210,000 alcohol abusers followed up for incidence.	No significant effect.
Monson and Lyon, 1975	Cohort. 1,382 alcoholics followed up for mortality.	Significant increase in risk with alcoholism (RR = 3.1).
Spalajkovic, 1976	Case-control. 200 male cases, 200 controls. Drinkers compared to non-drinkers.	Significant increase in risk in drinkers (RR = 11.2), not adjusted for smoking.
Wynder et al., 1976	Case-control. 314 cases, 684 controls. Three drinking categories.	Significant increase in risk in heavy drinkers (RR = 2.3 for highest vs lowest category.
Williams and Horm, 1977	Case-control. 119 cases, 5,566 controls. Lifetime consumption in three categories.	Significantly elevated risk with high consumption among males (RR = 2.75 for highest vs lowest category, adjusted for smoking).
Hinds et al., 1979	Case-control. 47 cases, 47 controls. Four daily consumption categories.	Significant increase in risk for heavy drinkers. Effect stronger among smokers.
Robinette et al., 1979	Cohort. 4,401 alcoholics and 4,401 controls followed up for mortality.	No significant effect.
Jensen, 1979	Cohort. 14,313 male brewery workers followed up for incidence.	Significantly elevated risk for brewery workers (RR = 2.2).
Burch et al., 1981	Case-control. 184 cases, 184 controls. Three daily consumption categories.	Significant increase in risk among drinkers, adjusted for smoking (RR = 4.0).
Herity et al., 1981	Case-control. 59 cases, 200 controls. Three consumption categories.	Increased risk with high intake (RR = 3.2, unadjusted), significance not known.

Table 6.8: (*Continued*)

Study	Design and Methods	Summary of qualitative results
Schmidt and Popham, 1981	Cohort. 9,889 male alcoholics followed up for mortality.	Significantly higher risk in alcoholics (RR = 4.5), compared to a population with similar smoking habits.
Elwood et al., 1984	Case-control. 154 cases, 154 controls. Five weekly consumption categories.	Significantly elevated risk extrinsic larynx cancer in heavy drinkers (RR = 6.4 for highest category), adjusted for smoking.
Olsen et al., 1985	Case-control. 326 cases, 1,134 controls. Includes hypopharyngeal cancer. Four weekly consumption categories.	Increased risk with high consumption (RR = 4.1 in highest category), adjusted for smoking.
Brugere et al., 1986	Case-control. 466 cases, 2,000 controls. Four consumption categories.	Significantly increased risk, varying by subsite, for high consumption, adjusted for smoking.
Zagraniski et al., 1986	Case-control. 87 cases, 153 controls. Drinkers compared to non-drinkers.	Significantly higher risk for drinkers (RR = 4.2), adjusted for smoking.
De Stefani et al., 1987	Case-control. 1,076 male cases, 290 hospital controls. Four daily consumption categories.	Significantly higher risk for heavy drinkers (RR = 9.3), adjusted for smoking.
Brown et al., 1988	Case-control. 183, male cases, 250 controls. Drinkers compared.	Non-significant increase in risk among drinkers (RR = 2.1), to non-drinkers.
Guenel et al., 1988	Case-control. 411 cases, 4,135 controls. Four consumption categories.	Significant increase in risk with higher consumption, adjusted for smoking.
Tuyns et al., 1988	Case-control. 727 cases, 3,057 controls. Five consumption categories	Significantly higher risk, varying by subsite, with consumption, adjusted for smoking.

prospective assessment of consumption and risk, taking smoking into account. The case-control studies, however, give strong evidence that alcohol does increase the risk of laryngeal cancer in addition to the effect of smoking.

6.2.2 Partial quantitative overview

Alcohol as a binary risk factor. Table 6.9 shows relative risks for drinkers compared to non-drinkers in five studies supplying the information, and the combined relative risk estimate. Although the smoking-adjusted combined

Table 6.9: Relative risks of laryngeal cancer for drinkers compared to non-drinkers

Study	RR	(95% CI)	Significance
Wynder et al., 1956*	1.34	(0.44, 4.02)	n.s.
Williams and Horm, 1977	2.87	(1.96, 4.20)	p<0.001
Zagraniski et al., 1986*	4.20	(1.19, 14.71)	p<0.05
De Stefani et al., 1987	6.09	(2.56, 14.44)	p<0.001
Brown et al., 1988	2.10	(0.89, 4.90)	0.1>p>0.05
All studies	2.92	(2.16, 3.94)	p<0.001
No significant heterogeneity among studies			
Studies adjusted for smoking	2.20	(0.96, 5.03)	0.1>p>0.05
No significant heterogeneity among studies			

*Adjusted for smoking.

effect falls short of formal significance at 5% level, there is almost certainly an effect of alcohol in addition to that of smoking, the non-significance being attributable to lack of power when analysis is restricted to two studies.

Dose-response. Dose-response was assessed by the trend in the log-odds ratio with increasing alcohol consumption in ml/day of ethanol, estimated by logistic regression. After the trends were estimated, they were combined. Results are shown in Table 6.10. Although there is significant heterogeneity among studies, the effects are all in the same direction (increasing risk with increasing consumption). The smoking-adjusted estimate is almost identical to the crude estimate. The trend of 0.0128 is equivalent to a 31% increase in risk associated with an increased consumption of one pint of beer per day.

Table 6.10: Trends in the log-odds ratio for laryngeal cancer with increasing alcohol consumption in ml/day

Study	Trend	Standard error	Significance
Wynder et al., 1976*	0.0056	0.0014	p<0.001
Hinds et al., 1979	0.0166	0.0052	p<0.01
Elwood et al., 1984	0.0127	0.0025	p<0.001
Olsen et al., 1985*	0.0223	0.0044	p<0.001
Guenel et al., 1988*	0.0154	0.0009	p<0.001
All studies	0.0129	0.0007	p<0.001
Significant heterogeneity among studies, p<0.001			
Studies adjusted for smoking	0.0128	0.0008	p<0.001
Significant heterogeneity among studies, p<0.001			

*Adjusted for smoking.

6.2.3 Is there a biological relationship?

That alcohol increases the risk of laryngeal cancer seems to be an inevitable conclusion of the above. How this happens biologically is not established. There is a school of thought that the action of alcohol on this site is almost entirely an exacerbation of the effect of smoking by irritation of the tissue and by acting as a solvent for tobacco carcinogens (Schmidt and Popham, 1981; Peto, 1985). However, an increased risk has been observed in association with drinking in non-smokers (Elwood et al., 1984) and light smokers (Olsen et al., 1985; Guenel et al., 1988), so this does not fully explain the effect of alcohol. Alcohol itself may be carcinogenic at this site, or if not, co-carcinogens in the beverages may be active on laryngeal tissue (although there is no evidence of a beverage-specific effect), or the effect may be due to alcohol-induced nutritional impairment (Robinette et al., 1979). It is likely that there is a causal relationship, but the nature of that relationship is probably an unknown combination of the mechanisms described above.

6.2.4 Attributable risk

If we first consider all drinking, the proportions of drinkers in England and Wales are estimated as 95% of men and 92% of women (Goddard and Ikin, 1989). These combine with the overall unadjusted relative risk estimate of 2.92 in Table 6.9 to give attributable risks of 65% in men and 64% in women. In 1987, there were 678 deaths among males and 188 among females from cancer of the larynx (OPCS, 1989). This gives a potential total avoidance of 561 (males and females combined) deaths per year from this disease which might be brought about by eliminating all drinking. If we take the smoking-adjusted relative risk of 2.20, we estimate the saving as 460 deaths per year (attributable risks are 53% in males and 52% in females). While this seems a modest saving for a high relative risk, it should be remembered that this disease is not generally fatal. In 1984, there were 1,488 male and 311 female registrations of laryngeal cancer in England and Wales (OPCS, 1988). Using the smoking-adjusted attributable risks, we should expect to prevent 950 cases (not deaths) per year by eliminating all drinking. Now consider the effect of reducing average consumption. From data in Goddard and Ikin (1989), we can estimate median daily consumption in England and Wales as 21 ml/day in men and 5 ml/day in women. If we propose to cut these by half, the combined trend estimate (adjusted for smoking) in Table 6.6 would predict risk reductions of 13% in men and 3% in women, leading to an avoidance of 94 deaths and 203 cases per year.

6.3 Alcohol and cancer of the oesophagus

6.3.1 Published research

Thirty-one studies were reviewed. Details are shown in Table 6.11.

Table 6.11: Design and brief summaries of results of studies of cancer of the oesophagus reviewed

Study	Design	Qualitative results
Wynder and Bross, 1961	Case-control. 150 male cases, 150 hospital controls. Drinks per day and beverage-specific analysis.	No significant differences in quantity, type or age of starting to drink, but cases drank more than controls. No adjustment for smoking.
Sundby, 1967*	Cohort. Alcoholics followed up for death from oesophageal cancer.	Significantly increased risk associated with alcoholism (RR = 4.1).
Martinez, 1969	Case-control. 179 male cases, 537 controls from hospital (1 per case) and community (2 per case). Units per day and beverage-specific analysis.	Cases drank more total alcohol (RR = 4.91 for 5+ to none), mixed drinks more often and tended to dilute drinks less often.
Bradshaw and Schonland, 1969	Case-control. 98 male cases, 341 non-malignant hospital controls. Ever-drinkers versus never.	No significant difference in amount of alcohol consumed but cases were more likely to drink local concoctions.
Bjelke, 1973	Case-control. 52 cases, 1,657 controls. Four consumption categories for beer, wine and spirits.	Significantly increased risk for high beer (RR = 4.4) and high spirits (RR = 2.1) consumption.
Bradshaw and Schonland, 1974	Case-control. 196 cases, 1,064 non-malignant hospital controls.	After adjustment for smoking, no significant differences in alcohol consumed.
De Jong et al., 1974	Case-control. 174 cases, 665 hospital controls. Beverage-specific analysis.	Male cases drank samsu, the local beverage, more often (RR = 2.87 for daily vs never). Female cases drank samsu more often (RR = 5.16 ever vs never). Male cases drank more samsu when adjusted for smoking, diet, dialect, area and education.
Hakulinen et al., 1974	Cohort. 210,000 male alcoholics followed up for incidence.	Significantly increased risk (RR = 4.1) with alcoholism.
Monson and Lyon, 1975	Cohort. 1,382 (1,139 male) alcoholics followed up for mortality.	Non-significant increase in risk associated with alcoholism (RR = 1.9).
Adelstein and White, 1976	Cohort. 2,070 (1,595 male) alcoholics followed up for mortality.	Significantly increased risk associated with alcoholism (RR = 3.9).
Williams and Horm, 1977	Case-control. 72 (49 male) cases, 5,566 (2,102 male) controls. Lifetime consumption of total alcohol, beer, wine and spirits.	Significantly increased risk with high alcohol consumption in females (RR = 8.1) adjusting for smoking, age and race.

Table 6.11: (Continued)

Study	Design	Qualitative results
Tuyns et al., 1977*	Case-control. 200 cases, 778 controls (all male). Six consumption categories.	Significant effect of consumption on risk (RR = 18.3 for highest category compared with lowest).
Dean et al., 1979	Cohort. Brewery workers (male) followed up (3–4000 in each of four five-year periods) for mortality.	No significant difference in risk from general population.
Hirayama, 1979*	Cohort. Study size not known.	RR = 1.7 and 2.0 for whisky and shochu drinking respectively – no details.
Robinette et al., 1979	Cohort. 4,401 alcoholics and 4,401 controls (males) followed up for mortality.	Non-significant increase in risk for alcoholics (RR = 2.0).
Tuyns et al., 1979	Case-control. 312 male cases, 869 hospital controls. Grams of ethanol/day and beverage-specific analysis.	Significant increasing trend in risk with consumption, adjusted for smoking. Strong drinks have greatest effect.
Jensen, 1980	Cohort. 14,313 male brewery workers followed up for incidence.	Significantly increased risk associated with brewery working (RR = 2.1).
Schmidt and Popham, 1981	Cohort. 9,889 male alcoholics followed up for mortality.	Significant increased risk associated with alcoholism (RR = 2.3), controlling indirectly for smoking.
Pottern et al., 1981	Case-control. 120 black male autopsy cases, 250 autopsy controls. Ethanol/day (five categories) and beverage-specific analysis.	Cases drank significantly more total alcohol than controls (RR = 7.5 for highest vs lowest category). Effects stronger for hard liquor than beer or wine. Not adjusted for tobacco.
Vassallo et al., 1985	Case-control. 226 cases, 469 hospital controls. Alcohol in cubic cm/day (3 categories).	Cases drank significantly more than controls (RR = 7.6 for 100+ cubic cm vs none) adjusted for smoking.
Victoria et al., 1987	Case-control. 171 cases, 342 hospital controls. Lifetime alcohol intake, cachaca intake and duration of drinking.	Amount of cachaca (g/day) and duration of drinking were significant adjusted for area, smoking and diet, (RR = 7.6 for high vs low intake).
MacDonald and MacDonald, 1987	Case-control. 129 cases, 212 controls with stomach cancer.	No significant differences observed.
Mandard et al., 1987	Case-control. 38 male cases, 37 healthy controls. Ethanol in g/day.	No significant differences after adjusting for tobacco.

Table 6.11: (*Continued*)

Study	Design	Qualitative results
Segal et al., 1988	Case-control. 200 cases, 391 controls. Beverage-specific and total alcohol (g/day) studied.	Cases drank significantly more total alcohol and traditional beer than controls. Male cases drank more spirits. Adjusted for smoking.
Yu et al., 1988	Case-control. 275 cases, 275 healthy controls. Ethanol (g/day) and beverage-specific analysis.	Cases drank significantly more total alcohol (RR = 10.3 for high intake vs none), beer, wine and spirits than controls.
Nakachi et al., 1988	Case-control. 343 autopsy cases, 343 healthy controls. Lifetime consumption estimated.	Male cases drank more than controls (RR = 2.6 for high vs low intake). Unadjusted for smoking.
Notani, 1988	Case-control. 236 cases, 215 hospital and 177 healthy controls. Total alcohol.	No significant association with alcohol consumption.
Prior, 1988	Cohort. 1,110 alcoholics followed up for incidence.	Significantly increased risk associated with alcoholism (RR = 3.8).
Brown et al., 1988	Case-control. 74 male cases, 157 hospital controls. Ethanol (oz/day) and beverage-specific analysis. Contemporaneous mortality study.	Cases drank hard liquor and moonshine significantly more often than controls (RR = 2.6) adjusted for tobacco. Heavy drinkers (>9oz/day) were more likely to die.
La Vecchia and Negri, 1989	Case-control. 250 cases, 1,089 hospital controls. Alcohol in drinks/day among non-smokers.	Cases drank significantly more than controls (RR = 3.6 for 8 drinks/day vs none).
Hebert and Kabat, 1989	Case-control. 303 cases, 453 controls. Alcohol in oz/day among current smokers.	Both male (RR = 2.2 for 1+ oz/day vs none) and female (RR = 2.8) cases drank significantly more than controls, adjusted for education, religion, race and amount of tobacco smoked.

*Publication not available, results obtained from IARC monograph.

Twenty-one studies were of case-control design. Of these, fifteen (Martinez, 1969; Bjelke, 1973; De Jong et al., 1974; Williams and Horm, 1977; Tuyns et al., 1977; Tuyns et al., 1979; Pottern et al., 1981; Vassallo et al., 1985; Victoria et al., 1987; Segal et al., 1988; Yu et al., 1988; Nakachi et al., 1988; Brown et al., 1988; La Vecchia and Negri, 1989; Hebert and Kabat, 1989) reported significant effects of consumption on risk, all in the direction of predisposing to disease. Of these, only three (Bjelke, 1973;

Table 6.12: Relative risks of oesophageal cancer for drinkers compared to non-drinkers

Study	RR	95% CI	Significance
Wynder and Bross, 1961	2.39	(0.60, 9.42)	n.s.
Martinez, 1969*	1.52	(0.94, 2.46)	0.1<p<0.05
Bradshaw and Schonland, 1969	1.55	(0.76, 3.15)	n.s.
Bradshaw and Schonland, 1974*	1.04	(0.56, 1.94)	n.s.
Williams and Horm, 1977	1.86	(1.15, 3.01)	p<0.05
Tuyns et al., 1979	5.21	(3.22, 8.42)	p<0.001
Pottern et al., 1981	5.87	(2.24, 15.34)	p<0.001
Vassallo et al., 1985	4.31	(2.66, 6.96)	p<0.001
Victoria et al., 1987	3.49	(2.35, 5.17)	p<0.001
MacDonald and MacDonald, 1987	1.55	(0.81, 2.97)	n.s.
Yu et al., 1988	4.57	(1.65, 12.66)	p<0.01
Notani, 1988*	1.30	(0.72, 2.34)	n.s.
Brown et al., 1988	5.26	(1.54, 17.89)	p<0.01
La Vecchia and Negri, 1989*	1.22	(0.57, 2.61)	n.s.
Herbert and Kabat, 1989	2.36	(1.68, 3.32)	p<0.001
All studies	2.41	(2.08, 2.79)	p<0.001
Significant heterogeneity among studies p<0.001			
Studies adjusting for smoking	1.30	(0.96, 1.75)	0.1<p<0.05
No significant heterogeneity			

*Directly or indirectly adjusted for smoking.

Pottern et al., 1981; Nakachi et al., 1988) incorporated no control for smoking.

Seven studies followed up cohorts of alcoholics. Five (Sundby, 1967; Hakulinen et al., 1974; Adelstein and White, 1976; Schmidt and Popham, 1981; Prior, 1988) found significantly increased risks in association with alcoholism. Of these, two (Sundby, 1967; Schmidt and Popham, 1981) indirectly adjusted for smoking by choice of comparison group. Two studies followed up cohorts of brewery workers. One (Jensen, 1980) found a significantly increased risk associated with this group. Only one study (Hirayama, 1979) prospectively assessed the effect of consumption on risk. After adjustment for smoking, relative risks of 1.7 and 2.0 were associated with whisky and shochu-drinking respectively (see IARC monograph).

Thus there is a large body of research on the subject, and with several positive results after adjustment for smoking, the qualitative indication is that alcohol-drinking does increase risk in addition to the effect of tobacco-smoking.

6.3.2 Partial quantitative overview

Alcohol as a binary risk factor. Table 6.12 shows relative risks observed for drinkers as compared with non-drinkers. The relative risk for all studies

Table 6.13: Trends in the log odds ratio relative risk of oesophageal cancer estimate with alcohol consumption in ml/day of ethanol

Study	Trend	SE	Significance
Wynder and Bross, 1961	0.0097	0.0019	$p<0.001$
Martinez, 1969	0.0159	0.0034	$p<0.001$
Tuyns et al., 1979	0.0199	0.0014	$p<0.001$
Pottern et al., 1981	0.0016	0.0005	$p<0.01$
Vassallo et al., 1985	0.0533	0.0055	$p<0.001$
Mandard et al., 1987	−0.0139	0.0063	$p<0.05$
Yu et al., 1988	0.0088	0.0023	$p<0.001$
La Vecchia and Negri, 1989	0.0040	0.0047	$p = 0.3$
Hebert and Kabat, 1989	0.0065	0.0011	$p<0.001$
All studies	0.0049	0.0004	$p<0.001$

Significant heterogeneity among studies, $p<0.001$

combined is shown at the foot of the table. The combined relative risk using all studies is 2.41, but that from the four studies from which smoking-adjusted relative risks were obtainable was 1.30. Further, there is significant heterogeneity among all studies, but not among those with adjustment for smoking.

Dose-response. Trends in the log-odds ratio for those studies reporting sufficient information for this to be assessed are shown in Table 6.13, with the combined trend. These trends are unadjusted for smoking apart from the study by Martinez (1969), in which there was matching for smoking. The combined trend is 0.0049 per ml/day. This corresponds to a relative risk of 1.1 in association with an increased consumption of one pint of beer per day. Although there is significant heterogeneity among studies, the direction of the trend is the same in all studies except that of Mandard et al. (1987), which had only 38 cases.

6.3.3 Is there a biological relationship?

There are a number of possible mechanisms for alcohol-drinking to enhance oesophageal cancer risk. One is as a transport agent, whereby alcohol assists the transfer of carcinogens (from tobacco for example) through the oesophageal mucosa. It seems unlikely that this is the sole mechanism, since many of the studies have found an effect of alcohol in addition to that of tobacco, and alcohol had an effect among non-smokers in La Vecchia and Negri's (1989) study. Another possibility is that alcohol acts as an irritant and thus accelerates epithelial cell turnover and hastens genetic damage. A third mechanism might be alcohol-induced nutritional imbalance, since high alcohol intakes can cause deficiencies in micronutrients even though dietary intakes are normal. It seems likely that alcohol acts in all three of these ways (Day et al., 1982). Alcohol should be regarded as at least an indirect contributor to risk, enhancing the effect of other carcinogens, and probably as a causal factor in its own right.

6.3.4 Attributable risk

The estimated proportions of drinkers in England and Wales are 95% in men and 92% in women (Goddard and Ikin, 1989). In combination with the combined relative risk of 2.41 for drinkers compared to non-drinkers in Table 6.12, this gives attributable risks of 57% in men and 56% in women. There were 2,851 deaths from cancer of the oesophagus in men in 1987 and 1,918 in women, in England and Wales (OPCS, 1989). This suggests that a total of 2,699 deaths per year could be avoided in England and Wales in both sexes combined, by eliminating all drinking. However, this does not take account of smoking. If we use the smoking-adjusted relative risk of 1.30, we obtain an attributable risk of 22% in men and women leading to an estimated 1,049 deaths per year avoided by eliminating all drinking. The latter seems more plausible.

If instead we consider reducing the amount consumed, we use the combined trend estimate in Table 6.13. The median daily consumption in England and Wales is approximately 21ml in men and 5ml in women (Goddard and Ikin, 1989). If we proposed to halve these figures, the trend estimate of 0.0049 would yield relative risks of 0.95 in men and 0.99 in women, thus decreasing the numbers of deaths by 5% and 1% respectively. This would yield an absolute saving of 162 deaths per year (143 in men and 19 in women). The disparity between the estimates for eliminating all drinking and for halving consumption may be due to a qualitative difference in risk between non-drinkers and drinkers, or to inaccuracy in measurement of actual amount consumed among drinkers, or a combination of both.

6.4 Alcohol and cancers of the stomach, colon and rectum

Here we review all major studies of alcohol consumption and risk of cancers of the stomach, colon and rectum. The latter two are treated together for purposes of overview.

6.4.1 Published research

For stomach cancer, 25 studies were reviewed. Twelve were case-control studies, six were cohort studies following up alcoholics specifically, two were cohort studies following up brewery workers who had higher beer consumption than the general population, four were cohort studies following up (approximately) general population subjects, and one was a descriptive study of a migrant population (details given in Table 6.14).

Of the case-control studies, five (Haenszel et al., 1972; Williams and Horm, 1977; Hoey et al., 1981; Jedrychowski et al., 1986; Hu et al., 1988) reported significant or suggestive positive associations of some aspect of consumption with risk. Of the studies on alcoholics, none reported any

Table 6.14: Studies assessing alcohol and stomach cancer risk

Study	Design and methods	Summary of results
Stocks, 1957	Case-control. 153 male cases, 4630 controls. Beer consumption.	No association with risk.
Wynder et al., 1963	Case-control. 521 (367 male) cases, 653 (401 male) controls. Drinks/day (6 categories).	No association with risk.
Higginson, 1966	Case-control. 93 (72 male) cases, 279 controls. Various non-quantitative categories.	Higher 'heavy period-ical' drinking in cases.
Sundby, 1967*	Cohort. Alcoholics followed up for mortality.	Slightly higher mort-ality rate among alcoholics (RR = 1.3).
Graham et al., 1972	Case-control. 228 (160 cases, 228 controls. 6 consumption categories.	No association with risk.
Haenszel et al., 1972	Case-control. 135 male Japanese cases, 270 hospital controls. Various beverages.	High risk (RR = 2.2) with high sake consumption (p < 0.05).
Bjelke, 1973	Case-control. 311 cases, 3,051 controls. Various beverages.	No significant effect on risk but possible effect of high beer consumption.
Hakulinen et al., 1974	Cohort. Roughly 4,370 alcoholics followed up for incidence.	No significant effect of alcoholism on risk (RR = 1.3).
Monson and Lyon, 1975	Cohort. 1,382 (1,139 male) alcoholics followed up for mortality.	No effect of alcoholism on risk (RR = 1.0).
Adelstein and White, 1976	Cohort. 2,070 (1,595 male) alcoholics followed up for mortality.	No effect of alcoholism on risk (RR = 0.8).
Williams and Horm, 1977	Case-control. 266 (158 male) cases, 5,468 (2,029 male) controls. Lifetime consumption and beverage-specific analysis.	No significant effect. Non-significant indication of effect of beer in women (RR = 2.0).
Dean et al., 1979	Cohort. Roughly 4,000 male brewery workers followed up for mortality.	No effect of brewery working on risk (RR = 0.8).
Robinette et al., 1979	Cohort. 4,401 alcoholics, 4,401 controls (all male) followed up for mortality.	No effect of alcoholism on risk (RR = 1.0).
Jensen, 1979	Cohort. 14,313 male brewery workers followed up for incidence.	No effect on risk (RR = 0.9).

Table 6.14: (*Continued*)

Study	Design and methods	Summary of results
Hoey et al., 1981	Case-control. 40 male cases, 168 hospital controls. Weekly alcohol consumption (4 categories). (RR = 6.9).	Significant increased risk with consumption of > 568 g/week
Klatsky et al., 1981	Cohort. 2,015 people in each of four consumption groups, followed up for mortality.	No effect of consumption on risk.
Schmidt and Popham, 1981.	Cohort. 9,889 male alcoholics followed up for mortality.	No effect of alcoholism on risk.
Tuyns et al., 1982	Case-control. 163 cases, 1,976 population controls. Ever versus never.	No effect of drinking (RR = 0.5 for drinkers compared to non-drinkers).
Gordon and Kannel, 1984	Cohort. 4,747 (2,106 male) population subjects followed up for mortality.	Significant association of high consumption with increased risk adjusted for smoking and other factors.
Pollack et al., 1984.	Cohort. 8,006 men followed up for incidence. Five consumption categories.	No effect of consumption on risk.
Trichopoulos et al., 1985	Case-control. 110 (57 male) cases, 100 (49 male) hospital controls. Four categories.	No significant effect of drinking on risk (RR = 1.5 for highest group compared with lowest).
Jedrychowski et al., 1986.	Case-control. 110 (70 male) cases, 110 controls. Drinking vodka before breakfast (yes/no).	Significant effect on risk (RR = 2.9 for drinking vodka before breakfast).
Kono et al., 1986	Cohort. 5,135 males followed up for mortality. Four consumption groups.	No effect on risk.
Ubukata et al., 1987	Migrant study. Drinking and cancer incidence compared between Koreans in Korea and in Japan.	Koreans in Japan drink more, but there was no substantial difference in rates.
Hu et al., 1988	Case-control. 241 (170 male) cases, 241 hospital controls. Two consumption categories.	Significant effect on risk (RR = 1.7 for high compared to low consumption).

*Publication unavailable, results from IARC monograph.

increased risk with alcoholism, nor did the two studies of brewery workers. Of those studies assessing the effect of consumption on risk prospectively among (approximately) population subjects, one (Gordon and Kannel, 1984) reported a significant increase in risk with high consumption. Since this study reported standardised logistic regression coefficients, relative risk estimates were not obtainable. The migrant study (Ubukata et al., 1987) did not show any indication of a relationship with risk.

For colorectal cancer, 25 studies were reviewed (with considerable overlap with the stomach cancer studies). Ten were case-control studies, six were cohort studies following up alcoholics, two were cohort studies of brewery workers, six were cohort studies of (approximately) general population members and one was the migrant study mentioned above (see Table 6.15).

Of the case-control studies, three (Wynder and Shigematsu, 1967; Tuyns et al., 1982; Potter and McMichael, 1986) found significant positive effects of some aspect of alcohol consumption on cancer at both sites. Three (Miller et al., 1983; Kabat et al., 1986; Kune et al., 1987) found significant results specifically associated with rectal cancer, all reporting increased risks in association with high beer consumption. Bjelke (1973) found a significant increase in colon cancer risk with high spirits consumption in men and a significant increase in rectal cancer risk with high beer consumption in both sexes. Williams and Horm (1977) found an increased risk of colon cancer with high alcohol consumption in males and an increased risk of rectal cancer with high alcohol consumption in females.

Of the cohort studies of alcoholics, two (Sundby, 1967; Robinette et al., 1979) found higher risks of rectal cancer to be associated with alcoholism. No other significant alcoholism-related results were observed. In the studies of brewery workers, Dean et al. (1979) found an increase in risk of rectal cancer among such workers, while Jensen et al. (1979) did not. Of the 'general population' cohort studies, Hirayama (1979) found a 50% increased risk of colon and small intestine cancers combined in association with daily drinking, Pollack et al. (1984) found a significant trend of increasing risk of rectal cancer with consumption (apparently mostly attributable to an effect of beer consumption) and Wu et al. (1987) found a significant increase in risk of colorectal cancer with high alcohol consumption. The migrant study of Ubukata et al. (1987) did not indicate any effect.

6.4.2 Partial quantitative overview

Alcohol as a binary risk factor. For stomach cancer, Table 6.16 shows relative risks for drinkers versus non-drinkers in those studies reporting the required information, and for all such studies combined. All in all, a significant effect is observed with drinkers having a relative risk of 1.17.

Table 6.17 shows the corresponding results for colorectal cancer. A similar combined effect is observed, with a relative risk of 1.21 for drinkers

Table 6.15: Studies assessing alcohol consumption and colorectal cancer risk

Study	Design and methods	Summary of results
Stocks, 1957*	Case-control. 166 male cases, 4,630 male controls. Colon and rectum with beer consumption.	Non-significant increase in risk with daily beer-drinking (RR = 1.4).
Higginson, 1966	Case-control. 340 male cases, 1,020 hospital controls. Colon and rectum.	No difference in consumption between cases and controls.
Sundby, 1967*	Cohort. Alcoholics followed up for cancers at both sites.	Increased risk of rectal cancer (RR = 1.9) but not colon (RR = 1.0).
Wynder and Shigematsu, 1967	Case-control. Both sites. 492 (288 colon) cases, 273 controls. Five consumption categories.	Rectal cancer significantly associated with high consumption. Both associated with high beer consumption.
Bjelke, 1973	Case-control. Both sites. 651 (421 colon) cases, 3,051 controls. Frequency of consumption by beverage.	Significant associations of colon cancer with spirits consumption positive for men, negative for women. Significant positive association of rectal cancer and beer for both sexes combined.
Hakulinen et al., 1974.	Cohort. Roughly 210,000 male alcoholics followed up for colon cancer incidence.	No significant effect of alcoholism on risk.
Monson and Lyon, 1975	Cohort. 1,382 (1,139 male) alcoholics followed up for colorectal cancer mortality.	No significant effect of alcoholism on risk (RR = 0.6).
Adelstein and White, 1976	Cohort. 2,070 (1,595 male) alcoholics followed up for intestinal and rectal cancer mortality.	No significant effect of alcoholism on risk (RR = 1.3 for intestine, RR = 0.9 for rectum).
Williams and Horm, 1977.	Case-control. Both sites. 1,061 (722 colon) cases, 4,673 controls. Lifetime consumption by beverage.	Significant increased risk of colon cancer with high consumption in males (RR = 1.5) and of rectal cancer in females (RR = 2.0). Adjusted for age, race and smoking.
Dean et al., 1979	Cohort. Male brewery workers followed up for colon and rectal cancer mortality.	Significant increased risk of rectal cancer (RR = 1.6).

Table 6.15: (*Continued*)

Study	Design and methods	Summary of results
Hirayama, 1979	Cohort. Details not known.	Daily drinking associated with 50% higher risk of intestinal cancer.
Jensen, 1979	Cohort. 14,313 male brewery workers followed up for incidence of colon and rectum cancers.	No association with risk.
Robinette et al., 1979.	Cohort. 4,401 alcoholics and 4,401 controls (all male) followed up for mortality from colon and rectal cancers.	Non-significant effect of alcoholism with rectal cancer risk (RR = 3.3).
Klatsky et al., 1981	Cohort. 2,015 subjects in each of four drinking categories followed up for colorectal cancer mortality.	No effect of consumption on risk.
Schmidt and Popham, 1981	Cohort. 9,889 male alcoholics followed up for mortality from colon and rectal cancers.	No effect of alcoholism on risk at either site.
Tuyns et al., 1982	Case-control. 340 (142 colon) cases, 1,976 population controls. Ever versus never.	Non-significant increased risk at each site (RR = 1.4 for colon, RR = 1.6 for rectum).
Miller et al., 1983	Case-control. 542 (348 colon) cases, 542 population controls, 535 hospital controls. Three beer categories and total alcohol analysed.	No significant effect of consumption after adjustment for diet. Increased risk of rectal cancer with high beer consumption for females only.
Gordon and Kannal, 1984	Cohort. 4,747 healthy subjects followed up for colon cancer mortality.	No effect of alcohol consumption on risk.
Pollack et al., 1984	Cohort. 8,006 healthy male subjects followed up for incidence of colon and rectal cancer. Five consumption categories.	Significant trend of risk of rectal cancer with consumption. Effect strongest with beer consumption.
Kabat et al., 1986	Case-control. 218 cases rectal cancer, 585 hospital controls.	Significant increase in risk with high beer consumption in males.
Kono et al., 1986	Cohort. 5,135 healthy males followed up for mortality from colorectal cancer.	No significant effect on risk.

Table 6.15: (*Continued*)

Study	Design and methods	Summary of results
Potter and McMichael, 1986	Case-control. 419 (220 colon) cases. Trends in risk by drinks per week, by beverage.	Significant increase in risk for spirit consumption for male colon and rectal cancer and female colon cancer.
Kune et al., 1987*	Case-control. Both sites. 715 cases, 727 controls. Risk by quintiles of beer intake.	Significant increase in rectal cancer with high beer consumption among males.
Wu et al., 1987	Cohort. 11,888 elderly people followed up for colorectal cancer. Three consumption categories.	Significant increase in risk with consumption in males.
Ubukata et al., 1987	Migrant study. Colon and rectal cancer incidence, and drinking habits of Koreans in Japan and Korea.	More drinkers among Koreans in Japan, but colon and rectal cancer incidence similar

*Publication unavailable, results from IARC monograph.

There is, however, significant heterogeneity among studies ($p < 0.01$), so this result should be interpreted with caution.

Dose-response. Trends of risk with increasing consumption were estimated within each study presenting results in sufficient detail in quantitative categories. These trends were then combined as described above.

Table 6.18 shows the results for stomach cancer, in terms of trend in the log-odds ratio per ml/day of ethanol. The combined estimate is not significant and there is significant heterogeneity among studies ($p < 0.001$). The combined estimate of 0.0025 per ml/day is equivalent to a 6% increase

Table 6.16: Relative risks of stomach cancer for drinkers as compared to non-drinkers

Study	RR	(95% CI)	Significance
Wynder et al., 1963	1.18	(0.87, 1.59)	n.s.
Higginson, 1966	1.03	(0.62, 1.72)	n.s.
Graham et al., 1972	1.02	(0.66, 1.59)	n.s.
Haenszel et al., 1972	1.32	(1.04, 1.67)	$p < 0.05$
Williams and Horm, 1977	1.18	(0.90, 1.55)	n.s.
Klatsky et al., 1981	1.11	(0.30, 4.04)	n.s.
Tuyns et al., 1982	0.54	(0.16, 1.80)	n.s.
Kono et al., 1986	0.98	(0.62, 1.53)	n.s.
All studies	1.17	(1.02, 1.33)	$p < 0.05$

No significant heterogeneity among studies

Table 6.17: Relative risks of colorectal cancer for drinkers versus non-drinkers

Study	RR	(95% CI)	Significance
Higginson, 1966	0.99	(0.76, 1.28)	n.s.
Wynder and Shigematsu, 1967	0.77	(0.54, 1.07)	n.s.
Williams and Horm, 1977	1.36	(1.17, 1.58)	p<0.001
Klatsky et al., 1981	1.78	(0.51, 6.11)	n.s.
Tuyns et al., 1982	1.51	(1.09, 2.10)	p<0.05
Kono et al., 1986	1.03	(0.46, 2.24)	n.s.
All studies	1.21	(1.08, 1.36)	p<0.001

Significant heterogeneity among studies, p<0.01

in risk with increased consumption of one pint of beer per day (21ml ethanol).

Table 6.19 shows the corresponding results for colorectal cancer. The combined estimate is not significant and there is no significant heterogeneity among studies. The combined trend of 0.0031 is equivalent to a 7% increase in risk with increased consumption of one pint of beer per day.

6.4.3 Is there a biological relationship?

Considering cancer of the stomach first, alcohol is known to have various effects on the stomach, although not necessarily carcinogenic effects. Examples are acute and chronic effects on acid secretion and predisposition to gastritis and gastric bleeding (IARC, 1988). This damage caused by alcohol may make the site more vulnerable to other carcinogens (Williams and Horm, 1977), or it may directly act as a carcinogen, although there is a high level of dilution of alcohol by the time it is in the stomach. In view of the generally negative results of individual studies, the general consensus is that there is no direct biological link of alcohol consumption and stomach cancer (IARC, 1988).

It is generally believed to be more likely that a biological relationship

Table 6.18: Trends in the log-odds ratio estimate of relative risk of stomach cancer with increasing alcohol consumption (ml/day)

Study	Trend	SE	Significance
Wynder et al., 1963	−0.0012	0.0020	n.s.
Hoey et al., 1981	0.0193	0.0040	p<0.001
Klatsky et al., 1981	0.0025	0.0060	n.s.
Kono et al., 1986	−0.0017	0.0037	n.s.
Hu et al., 1988	0.0372	0.0136	p<0.01
All studies	0.0025	0.0015	n.s.

Significant heterogeneity among studies p<0.001

Table 6.19: Trends in the log-odds ratio estimate of relative risk of colorectal cancer with increasing alcohol consumption (ml/day)

Study	Trend	SE	Significance
Wynder and Shigematsu, 1967	0.0035	0.0022	n.s.
Klatsky et al., 1981	−0.0008	0.0051	n.s.
Kono et al., 1986	0.0057	0.0068	n.s.
All studies	0.0031	0.0019	n.s.

No significant heterogeneity among studies

exists between colorectal cancer and alcohol consumption. A possible indirect effect is via diet, in that a high alcohol consumption is often associated with nutritional deficiencies. Dean et al. (1979) suggest confounding with fibre intake. Ubukata et al. (1987) suggest fat intake may be responsible. Wu et al. (1987) suggest that alcohol's effect of decreasing cholesterol saturation of bile by increasing bile acid concentration may in turn affect the formation of faecal carcinogens. Another possibility is damage to the intestinal mucosa, which in turn leads to increased susceptibility to carcinogens, as suggested for stomach above.

There is some evidence for an effect of consumption on rectal cancer alone, and in turn that this effect is specific to beer-drinking. It is not clear how this would occur biologically.

6.4.4 Attributable risk

For stomach cancer, the estimated proportions of drinkers in England and Wales of 95% of men and 92% of women (Goddard and Ikin, 1989) give approximate attributable risks of 14% in both men and women, using the combined relative risk of 1.17 in Table 6.16. This is the estimated proportion of cases due to all drinking. This amounts to a saving of 1,331 stomach fatalities per year, by eliminating all drinking (14% of 9,509 deaths per year – see OPCS, 1989). If instead we consider bringing down the average amount consumed by a realistic figure, we find a much more modest predicted effect. Goddard and Ikin's (1989) Table 2.12 suggests median consumptions of 21ml of ethanol per day in men and 5ml per day in women. The combined trend estimate in Table 6.18 in combination with halving these consumption levels yields decreases in risk of 3% in men and 1% in women. Since there were 5,723 deaths in 1987 in men and 3,786 in women (OPCS, 1989), this amounts to a saving of 210 deaths per year. Since the combined trend estimate was not significant, and there was significant heterogeneity among studies, even this modest benefit might not accrue. The fact that the effect of eliminating all drinking is greater than one might expect from the dose-response indicates that there is either a qualitative effect of drinking at all, or that the apparent effect is due to a confounding variable, possibly dietary.

For colorectal cancer, the corresponding attributable risks for all drinking are 17% in men and 16% in women. There were 8,228 colorectal cancer cases in men and 8,825 in women in 1987 (OPCS, 1989), in England and Wales. Together, these predict an absolute avoidance of 2,913 colorectal cancer deaths per year in England and Wales. There is substantial hetero-geneity among studies, so this result should be regarded as approximate. Using the result in Table 6.19, the corresponding saving from halving alcohol consumption in males and females would be 332 deaths per year in England and Wales. Again, since the combined trend estimate is not significant, even this saving is not guaranteed. As in the case of stomach cancer, the absence or small magnitude of the dose-response effect makes the effect of drinking at all difficult to interpret. It should be borne in mind that the effect may really be due to a dietary correlate.

6.5 Alcohol and lung cancer

6.5.1 Published research

Studies (24 in all) addressing the problem are shown in Table 6.20, with a brief description of the design and results of each study. There are sixteen cohort studies (prospective), seven case-control studies (retrospective) and one descriptive study of a migrant population, Koreans in Japan (Ubukata et al., 1987).

Of the cohort studies, eight followed up a group of alcoholics and compared their lung cancer incidence or mortality with a control cohort or general population rates. Six of these (Pell and D'Alonzo, 1973; Hakulinen et al., 1974; Monson and Lyon, 1975; Adelstein and White, 1976; Robinette et al., 1979; Prior, 1988) made no adjustment for tobacco use, and two (Sundby, 1967; Schmidt and Popham, 1981) compared the alcoholics' rates with those of a population with similar smoking habits to those of the alcoholics under study. Neither of the two studies finding a significant association with increased lung cancer risk (Hakulinen et al., 1974; Prior, 1988) had any adjustment for smoking.

Two cohort studies followed up brewery workers whose intakes of beer were higher than those of the general population. One, in Denmark (Jensen, 1979), found a significantly increased risk, but concluded that this was probably due to confounding with socioeconomic status as the increased risk (RR = 1.16, not adjusting for tobacco use) was also observed in mineral water bottling workers. The other, in Ireland (Dean et al., 1979), found no excess risk among brewery workers.

The remaining six cohort studies (Hirayama, 1979; Klatsky et al., 1981; Kvale et al., 1983; Pollack et al., 1984; Gordon and Kannel, 1984; Kono et al., 1986) followed up groups with varying degrees of alcohol consumption.

Table 6.20: Summary of studies on alcohol and lung cancer reviewed

Study	Design and methods	Results in brief
Schwartz et al., 1962	Case-control. 1,159 cases, 1,196 controls all males. Mean daily intakes compared.	Cases' intakes significantly higher than controls. Significance much reduced by adjusting for smoking.
Sundby, 1967*	Cohort. Alcoholics followed up for lung cancer mortality.	19 deaths, 13.2 expected from roughly comparable population. Not significant.
Bradshaw and Schonland, 1969	Case-control, 45 cases, 341 controls, all male.	More cases than controls drank. Result significant, but no adjustment for smoking.
Pell and D'Alonzo, 1973*	Cohort. Alcoholics and non-alcoholics followed up for lung cancer mortality.	5 deaths among alcoholics, 2 among controls. Not significant. No adjustment for smoking.
Hakulinen et al., 1974	Cohort. Male alcoholics followed up for lung cancer incidence.	233 lung cancers, 119.4 expected. Significant but no adjustment for smoking.
Monson and Lyon, 1975	Cohort. 1,382 male alcoholics followed up for lung cancer mortality.	19 lung cancer deaths, 14.1 expected. Not significant. No adjustment for smoking.
Adelstein and White, 1976	Cohort. 2,070 (1,595) alcoholics followed up for lung cancer mortality.	Significantly increased risk in females (8 deaths, 2.5 expected). No adjustment for smoking.
Williams and Horm, 1977	Case-control. 931 (737 male) cases, 5,566 (2,102 male) controls. Total life consumption studied.	Significantly increased risk with high consumption. Significance lost when adjusted for smoking.
Dean et al., 1979	Cohort. Male brewery workers (approx. 4,000) followed up for lung cancer mortality.	98 lung cancer deaths, 109.1 expected, controlling for socioeconomic status.
Hirayama, 1979*	Cohort. Study size not given.	No effect among smokers.
Jensen, 1979	Cohort. 14,313 male brewery workers followed up for lung cancer incidence.	287 cases, 247.9 expected. Authors suggest confounding with socioeconomic status.
Robinette et al., 1979	Cohort. 4,401 male alcoholics and 4,401 nasopharyngitis controls followed up for lung cancer mortality.	No significant effect. Controls may be at high risk of lung cancer.
Schmidt and Popham, 1981	Cohort, 9,889 alcoholics (male) followed up for lung cancer mortality.	89 deaths, 90.7 expected in population with similar smoking habits.

Table 6.20: (*Continued*)

Study	Design and methods	Results in brief
Klatsky et al., 1981	Cohort. 2,015 subjects (1,584 male) in each of four consumption groups followed up for lung cancer mortality.	Possible modest effect, but potential for residual confounding with smoking, despite approximate matching for smoking.
Herity et al., 1982	Case-control. 59 cases, 152 controls, all male.	No significant effect when adjusted for smoking.
Kvale et al., 1983	Cohort. 16,713 (13,785 male) healthy subjects followed up for lung cancer incidence.	Significantly increased risk with high consumption only among those with low vitamin A intakes.
Pollack et al., 1984	Cohort. 8,006 health males followed up for lung cancer incidence.	Significant trend of increasing risk with alcohol consumption after adjustment for smoking.
Gordon and Kannel, 1984	Cohort. 4,747 healthy subjects (2,106) males) followed up for lung cancer mortality.	Increased risk with high alcohol consumption. Disappears when adjusted for smoking.
Kono et al., 1986	Cohort. 5,135 males followed up for lung cancer mortality.	No significant effect of alcohol consumption.
Ubukatu et al., 1987	Migrant study. Lung cancer mortality and drinking in Koreans in Japan compared with Koreans in Korea.	Immigrants drink more and have higher lung cancer rates. No adjustment for smoking.
Holst et al., 1988	Case-control. 49 cases (37 male), 98 controls, sex-matched.	No significant difference between cases and controls by mean consumption.
Prior, 1988	Cohort. 1,110 alcoholics (876 males) followed up for lung cancer incidence.	Significantly increased risk in male alcoholics (44 cases, 19.2 expected). No adjustment for smoking.
Mettlin, 1989	Case-control. 569 cases (355) male) and 569 sex-matched controls.	No effect of alcohol consumption on risk, adjusting for smoking.
Pierce et al., 1989	Case-control. 71 cases, 71 controls, all male. Duration and weekly consumption compared.	Slightly higher weekly consumption, not significant.

*Publication not available, data from IARC monograph (1988).

Hirayama (1979) found no effect of consumption on risk among smokers, but did not quote a result for non-smokers. The other five studies incorporated adjustment for smoking, although the one finding a significant effect of consumption on risk (Pollack et al., 1984) did not quote sufficient data to assess the nature of the adjustment or the extent of residual confounding, the extent to which alcohol consumption is related to unmeasured smoking (see related report on bladder cancer). Kvale et al. (1983) found an increased risk with high consumption among those with low vitamin A intakes, but the main thrust of the study was the effect of vitamin A rather than drinking, so the published data on drinking are minimal and hence difficult to interpret. Klatsky et al. (1981) found a relative risk of 1.6 (non-significant) for those taking six or more drinks per day compared with non-drinkers, but noted the possibility of residual confounding with smoking. The remaining three studies found no significant effect when adjusted for smoking.

The migrant study (Ubukata et al., 1987) found that Koreans in Japan drink more than in Korea and have correspondingly higher lung cancer rates. The authors draw no inferences from this, as there is confounding with smoking and other lifestyle factors.

Of the seven case-control studies (Schwartz et al., 1962; Bradshaw and Schonland, 1969; Williams and Horm, 1977; Herity et al., 1982; Holst et al., 1988; Mettlin, 1989; Pierce et al., 1989), only two (Bradshaw and Schonland, 1969; Pierce et al., 1989) did not control for smoking or at least publish sufficient data for the reader to assess the likelihood of an effect of alcohol independent of smoking. Two studies found a significantly increased risk associated with alcohol consumption, Schwartz et al. (1962) finding the increase significant after adjustment for smoking and Bradshaw and Schonland (1969) not attempting to adjust.

If there can be said to be an overall impression of the above studies, it is a broadly negative one, with the positive results mostly in those studies which did not control for tobacco use. The absence of control for such a powerful confounder is a considerable hindrance to interpretation, as we shall see when we attempt a quantitative overview.

6.5.2 Partial quantitative overview

Risk among alcoholics. Table 6.21 shows relative risks and confidence intervals associated with alcoholism in the eight studies specifically following up alcoholics, and the combined results. The combined result from all studies shows a significantly increased risk (1.53) associated with alcoholism, but this is due mainly to two studies (Hakulinen et al., 1974; Prior, 1988), neither of which took account of smoking. There is significant heterogeneity of the effect from study to study, rendering the combined result difficult to interpret. When we combine the two studies which compared the alcoholics with people of similar smoking habits (Sundby, 1967; Schmidt and Popham, 1981), there is no longer any significant effect (RR = 1.05).

Dose response. In studies publishing sufficient data, trends in the log-odds ratio were estimated by consumption in litres of ethanol per week. Only three studies published the results in such a way that the data were

Table 6.21: Review and overview of lung cancer risk related to alcoholism

Study	Adjusted for smoking	Relative risk	95% confidence interval	Significance
Sundby, 1967	Indirectly	1.44	(0.91, 2.25)	n.s.*
Pell and D'Alonzo, 1973	No	2.00	(0.82, 4.79)	n.s.
Hakulinen et al., 1974	No	1.95	(1.71, 2.23)	p<0.001
Monson and Lyon, 1975	No	1.35	(0.85, 2.10)	n.s.
Adelstein and White, 1975	No	1.16	(0.86, 1.57)	n.s.
Robinette et al., 1979	No	1.06	(0.80, 1.41)	n.s.
Schmidt and Popham, 1981	Yes	0.98	(0.79, 1.21)	n.s.
Prior, 1988	No	2.24	(1.67, 3.02)	p<0.001
All studies		1.53	(1.39, 1.67)	p<0.001

Heterogeneity among studies, Chi-squared = 67.0 (7 df), p<0.001.
Two studies with control for smoking, combined RR = 1.05, 95% confidence interval (0.86, 1.27), n.s.
*n.s. = not significant

retrievable to perform this exercise, but they did all yield estimates with at least partial adjustment for smoking, in one case (Klatsky et al., 1981) by matching, in one (Herity et al., 1982) by presenting results in light and heavy smokers separately, and in one (Kono et al., 1986) by explicitly reporting the adjusted trend. Results are shown in Table 6.22. The overall

Table 6.22. Dose-response as measured by trends in log odds ratios for lung cancer with litres of ethanol consumed per week

Study	Number of cases	Trend (smoking-adjusted)	SE(trend)*	Significance
Klatsky et al., 1981	62	0.9436	0.3984	p<0.05
Herity et al., 1982	59	0.3425	0.5694	n.s.
Kono et al., 1986	74	−0.6455	0.6878	n.s.
All studies	195	0.5016	0.2912	n.s.

Heterogeneity among studies, Chi-squared = 6.43 (2 df), p<0.05.

*SE = standard error.

Table 6.23: Drinking as a binary risk factor for lung cancer (risk in drinkers compared to that in non-drinkers)

Study	Adjusted for smoking	Relative risk	95% confidence interval	Significance
Bradshaw and Schonland, 1969	No	3.78	(0.88, 16.10)	n.s.
Williams and Horm, 1977	No	1.33	(1.12, 1.57)	$p < 0.05$
Klatsky et al., 1981	Yes	0.96	(0.53, 1.72)	$p < 0.05$
Kono et al., 1986	No	0.55	(0.33, 0.90)	$p < 0.05$
All studies		1.20	(1.03, 1.41)	$p < 0.05$

Heterogeneity among studies, Chi-squared = 21.4 (3 df), $p < 0.001$

effect is not significant. Again there is significant heterogeneity among studies, the Kono et al. (1986) study yielding a negative trend and the others positive. This is probably due to the fact that adjustment for smoking in the other two studies is crude, leaving considerable scope for residual confounding.

Drinking as a binary risk factor. Four studies reported results in a form enabling a comparison of drinkers with non-drinkers (Bradshaw and Schonland, 1969; Williams and Horm, 1977; Klatsky et al., 1981; Kono et al., 1986). Of necessity, in all but the Klatsky et al. (1981) study, unadjusted data had to be used to obtain a relative risk estimate. Results are shown in Table 6.23. Although the overall result is significant there is heterogeneity among results yet again. The only relative risk adjusted for tobacco consumption is that of Klatsky et al., indicating no effect of drinking at all.

6.5.4 Is there a biological relationship?

In the IARC monograph (1988) on alcohol and cancer risk, it is stated 'In view of the lack of excess risk in case-control studies and the inconsistent results of cohort studies, there is no indication that drinking of alcoholic beverages has a causal role in lung cancer'. The present results seem to back up this conclusion, indicating that apparent effects of alcohol consumption on risk are largely due to confounding with smoking. The one possible biological role that alcohol may have is in interaction with vitamin A deficiency. If lack of vitamin A predisposes towards lung cancer, alcoholics may be at high risk due to dietary vitamin A deficiency and at a further increased risk because the excessive alcohol consumption leads to accelerated depletion of liver vitamin A. This might explain the higher risk observed among heavy drinkers with already low vitamin A intakes in

Kvale's study (1983). This hypothesis is also discussed by Prior (1988). This effect, however, would be confined to a small subset of the population, and in any case the evidence for it is tentative.

The results of Jensen (1979) suggest the possibility of an effect of beer-drinking in particular, or of a factor correlated with beer-drinking. This is not borne out by the study of Dublin brewery workers (Dean et al., 1979) or by the three case-control studies considering beverage-specific risks (Williams and Horm, 1977; Pollack et al., 1984; Mettlin, 1989).

6.5.5 Attributable risk

Relative risks can be converted to attributable risks, the percentage of cases avoidable by eliminating the risk factor, but, given the equivocal nature of the data, our conclusions must be tentative. The annual death rates in the United Kingdom from cancer of the trachea, bronchus and lung are 979 per million in males and 399 per million in females (OPCS, 1989). First, considering the attributable risk for alcoholism, we have the difficulty of defining alcoholism in order to achieve a prevalence estimate. Since an arbitrary decision has to be made, let us assume that the fairly heavy and very heavy consumers in Goddard and Ikin's (1989) survey can be considered alcoholics, i.e. 12% of men and 2% of women. The relative risk of 1.53, unadjusted for smoking, from Table 6.21 would yield an attributable risk of 6% for males and 1% for females, reducing the death rates to 920 per million in men and 395 per million in women, if we could eliminate alcoholism. This corresponds to saving 1,549 lives per year (in men and women in total). If we use the smoking-adjusted RR estimate of 1.05, we obtain attributable risks of 0.6% in males and 0.1% in women, amounting to a saving of 154 lives in all if alcoholism were eliminated. The fact that the relative risk is not significantly different from unity indicates that even this minor benefit might not be achieved.

Now consider the attributable risk from all drinking. Goddard and Ikin (1989) estimate the prevalence of drinkers as 95% of men and 92% of women. The estimated RR of 1.20 from the four studies combined in Table 6.23 would give attributable risks of 16% in men and in women. Thus, eliminating drinking altogether (admittedly hypothetical) would avoid 16% of lung cancer deaths in each sex, i.e. 5,485 lung cancer deaths per year. Unfortunately, if we take the estimate from the study of Klatsky et al. (1981), the one of these four which incorporates a control for smoking, the relative risk is 96%, yielding an attributable risk of zero, and leading to the conclusion that no lung cancer deaths would be avoided by eliminating drinking. In view of the strength of smoking as a risk factor and as a confounder with alcohol, the latter conclusion is the more likely one.

Now let us consider the dose-response trend. From the three studies in Table 6.22, we have a (non-significant) trend of 0.5016 in the log-odds ratio per litre of ethanol per week. This corresponds to a relative risk of 1.65 for those drinking a litre of alcohol a week relative to those drinking none (or for those drinking two litres relative to those drinking one litre). In England and Wales, median alcohol consumption is approximately 148ml per week in men and 32ml per week in women (Goddard and Ikin, 1989). Reducing the male intake to 50ml per week would bring about an overall reduction of 5% in risk avoiding 49 deaths per million per year (1,199 deaths in England and Wales as a whole). In females, a reduction of intake to 10ml per week would reduce risk by 1%, avoiding 4 deaths per million per year (103 in England and Wales). However, since there is significant hetero-geneity among studies, these figures cannot be regarded as definitive. Also, since the result is not significant, it may be that there would be no bene-fit at all in reducing drinking. The fact that the positive trend is only observed in the two studies with scope for substantial residual confounding with smoking indicates that the figure of 0.5016 is almost certainly an overestimate.

In conclusion, it is most likely that changes in alcohol consumption unaccompanied by changes in smoking habits are unlikely to bring about substantial benefits in terms of reduced deaths from lung cancer.

6.6 Alcohol and female breast cancer

6.6.1 Published Research

We review 29 studies in all, and their design and results are summarised in Table 6.24. The majority of the work has been published since 1980. Nineteen (66%) of the studies are of retrospective case-control design (Williams and Horm, 1977; Byers and Funch, 1982; Rosenberg et al., 1982; Begg et al., 1983; Medina et al., 1983; Paganini-Hill and Ross, 1983; Webster et al., 1983; Le et al., 1984; Talamini et al., 1984; La Vecchia et al., 1985; Katsouyanni et al., 1986; Harvey et al., 1987; La Vecchia et al., 1987; Nielsen et al., 1987; O'Connell et al., 1987; Adami et al., 1988; Harris et al., 1988; Rohan and McMichael, 1988; Young, 1989). Of these, twelve (Williams and Horm, 1977; Rosenberg et al., 1982; Begg et al., 1983; Le et al., 1984; Talamini et al., 1984; La Vecchia et al., 1985; Harvey et al., 1987; La Vecchia et al., 1987; Nielsen et al., 1987; O'Connell et al., 1987; Rohan and McMichael, 1988; Young, 1989) found a significant or almost signifi-cant predisposing effect of alcohol consumption (alcohol abuse in the case of Nielsen et al., 1987).

There were five cohort studies following up subjects considered to represent the general, healthy population (Hiatt and Bawol, 1984; Schatzkin et al., 1987; Willett et al., 1987; Hiatt et al., 1988a; Schatzkin et al., 1989b). All but one (Schatzkin et al., 1989b) found an increased risk to be associated with high alcohol consumption.

Two cohort studies followed up female alcoholics specifically (Adelstein

Table 6.24: Summary of studies of alcohol and breast cancer

Study	Design and methods	Results in brief
Adelstein and White, 1976	Cohort. 475 female alcoholics followed up for breast cancer mortality, compared with general population.	Significantly more breast cancer deaths than expected. 10 deaths (4.46 expected, p<0.05). No control for other variables.
Williams and Horm, 1977	Case-control. 1,118 cases, 2,070 controls. Lifetime alcohol exposure used and beverage-specific analysis.	Significant increase in risk with use of wines, spirits and total alcohol (p<0.01) adjusting for age, race and smoking.
Byers and Funch, 1982	Case-control. 1,314 cases 770 controls. Drinks per month used.	No effect adjusted for age.
Rosenberg et al., 1982	Case-control. 1,152 cases 519 controls with endo-metrial or ovarian cancer, 2,702 with non-malignant disease. Drinks/week and beverage-specific analysis.	Significantly more cases drank than non-malignant disease controls, adjusted for socioeconomic factors.
Begg et al., 1983	Case-control. 997 cases 730 hospital controls. Drinks/week used.	Almost significant increased risk (RR = 1.4) with >7 drinks/week, adjusted for age and smoking.
Medina et al., 1983	Case-control. 76 cases, 76 controls.	Increased risk among 'moderate' drinkers (RR = 2.8), unadjusted, not significant.
Paganini-Hill and Ross, 1983	Case-control. 239 cases, 239 healthy controls. Drinks/day used.	No effect observed. Unadjusted.
Webster et al., 1983	Case-control. 1,226 cases 1,279 healthy controls. Grams per week and beverage-specific analysis.	No effect observed. Adjusted for smoking, reproduction variables and body mass index.
Hiatt and Bawol, 1984	Cohort. 88,477 women from general population. Drinks/day used.	Effect of drinking 3 or more drinks/day (RR = 1.38, p<0.05) adjusted for body mass, reproduction variables and cholesterol.
Le et al., 1984	Case-control. 1,010 cases 1,950 hospital controls. Grams per week and beverage-specific analysis.	Significant increase in risk with wine (p<0.05) adjusted for history and job.

Table 6.24: (*Continued*)

Study	Design and methods	Results in brief
Talamini et al., 1984	Case-control. 368 cases, 373 hospital controls. Drinks/day of wine used.	Significant increase in risk with wine ($p<0.001$) adjusted for reproduction and diet factors.
La Vecchia et al., 1985	Case-control. 437 cases, 437 hospital controls. Beverage-specific analysis.	Significant increase in risk with wine ($p<0.05$). and total alcohol ($p<0.01$) RR = 2.1 for >3 drinks/day, adjusted for social and reproductive factors.
Harvey et al., 1987	Case-control. 1,524 cases, 1,896 healthy controls. Grams per week used.	Significant increase in risk with beer, spirits and total alcohol ($p<0.05$).
La Vecchia et al., 1987	Case-control. 1,108 cases, 1,281 hospital controls. Drinks/day used.	Significant increase in risk with total alcohol ($p<0.001$), adjusted for diet, reproductive and social factors. RR = 2.9 for >4 to none.
Nielsen et al., 1987	Autopsy case-control. 22 cases, 88 controls. Alcohol abuse used.	Significant increased risk (RR = 3.2, $p<0.05$) with alcohol abuse, not adjusted.
O'Connell et al., 1987)	Case-control. 276 cases, 1,519 healthy controls. Comparing <1 drink per week to 1 or more per week.	Almost significant effect (RR = 1.45, 95% CI (0.99, 2.12), adjusted for age, race and reproductive factors.
Schatzkin et al., 1987	Cohort. 7,188 women from general population. Grams per day of alcohol used.	Significant increased risk ($p<0.05$). RR = 2.0 for >4 to none, adjusted for social, dietary and reproductive factors.
Smith, 1987	Temporal study of incidence. Beverage-specific analysis.	Significant increased risk with wine. Not interpretable.
Ubutaka et al., 1987	Migrant study of incidence.	Increased risk with, consumption. Not adjusted.
Willett et al., 1987	Cohort. 89,538 nurses. Grams per day of alcohol used.	Significant increased risk with .14g/day ($p<0.01$, RR = 1.6) adjusted for reproductive factors.
Adami et al., 1988	Case-control. 422 cases, 527 healthy controls. Grams per day of alcohol and beverage-specific analysis.	No effect observed, adjusted for smoking, social and reproductive factors.

Table 6.24: (*Continued*)

Study	Design and methods	Results in brief
Harris et al., 1988	Case-control. 1,467 cases 10,178 hospital controls. Grams per day alcohol used.	No effect observed after adjusting for age, smoking, social factors.
Hiatt et al., 1988	Cohort. 58,347 women. Subsidiary case-control study. 303 cases, 5,835 controls. Drinks/day used.	Significant increased risk ($p < 0.05$). RR = 3.2 for >5 to none.
Prior, 1988	Cohort. 234 alcoholics.	2 cases observed. No adjustment.
Rohan and McMichael, 1988	Case-control. 451 cases, 451 healthy controls. Grams per day and beverage-specific analysis.	Significant increased risk ($p < 0.05$), adjusted for smoking, social, reproductive factors. RR = 1.57 for >9.3 to none.
Schatzkin et al., 1989a	International correlation study.	Significant positive marginal correlation, but loses its significance on adjusting for fat intake.
Schatzkin et al., 1989b	Cohort. 2,636 women. Grams per day of alcohol used.	No effect observed adjusted for smoking, social and reproductive factors.
Young, 1989	Case-control. 277 cases, 372 healthy controls, 433 hospital controls. Drinks/week used.	Significant increased risk ($p < 0.001$) with RR = 3.17 for >5 to none in 18–35-year-olds and RR = 2.67 for >5 to none in >35-year-olds.

and White, 1976; Prior, 1988). Adelstein and White found a significant increase in risk associated with alcoholism, while Prior (1988) did not.

In an international correlation study, Schatzkin et al. (1989a) found a significant association of national breast cancer incidence rates with national alcohol consumption, but this vanished when fat intake was taken into account. In a temporal study of incidence rates, Smith (1987) found that in years of heavy alcohol consumption in Western Australia, breast cancer incidence was higher than in years of lighter consumption. This result is not readily interpretable, as many other factors could contribute to both consumption and breast cancer incidence.

Similar problems of interpretation arise in Ubukata et al. (1987), where Koreans in Japan were found to drink more and have higher breast cancer incidence than Koreans in Korea. Evidence from these three papers can at best be considered circumstantial.

Both case-control and cohort studies will inevitably suffer from some bias of misclassification, which will tend to cause underestimation of effect, if the misclassification is equal for those with breast cancer and those without. When diet is included in the model, it too will be misclassified to some extent, and it should be borne in mind that misclassification of confounding variables can cause overestimation of the effect of interest (Duffy et al., 1989), although we might expect this latter bias to be relatively small.

Case-control studies in particular are prone to recall bias. This could be manifested as follows: suppose the cases, knowing that they are very ill, are more careful in remembering their alcohol consumption than controls who are healthy, or in a transient state of acute illness. There is also the related bias of increased frankness on the part of sick cases. While the case-control studies do not yield positive results more often than cohort studies, it may be that the relative risks estimated in some case-control studies are exaggerated by these biases. One such example might be the relative risk of 16.7 observed by Talamini et al. (1984) in association with drinking more than half a litre of wine per day.

6.6.2 Partial quantitative overview

Alcohol as a binary risk factor. Table 6.25 shows relative risks associated with drinking at all from those studies which yield the information needed to estimate them, and for all studies combined. These are of necessity unadjusted for other factors, but adjustment of the alcohol effect for other variables tended to make little difference in most studies (see below). The overall estimate is 1.20, but there is significant heterogeneity among studies, so this should not be overinterpreted.

Dose-response. For those studies reporting consumption in categories, median consumptions were estimated as the midpoint of each category and a trend in the log-odds ratio with increasing median consumption estimated by logistic regression (or log-linear modelling in the case of cohort studies). Results for individual studies, and all studies combined, are given in Table 6.26. The overall estimate is 0.59 per litre per week, corresponding to a relative risk of 1.80 for an increased consumption of 1 litre per week. Again, there is significant heterogeneity from study to study, so this should not be treated as definitive.

6.6.3 Is there a biological relationship?

Since most studies have found effects which did not seem to be attributable to confounding, it is reasonable to infer that alcohol and breast cancer risk are related. Before concluding that the relationship is causal, however, we should consider that there may be confounding with dietary factors as yet unidentified as risk factors for breast cancer.

Potential mechanisms for an effect of alcohol on breast cancer risk are not at all obvious. Possibilities are an indirect effect via liver damage in excessive drinkers, changes in the breast due to prolactin stimulation by

Table 6.25: Alcohol as a binary risk factor. Relative risks and confidence intervals associated with drinking at all compared to not drinking, in individual studies yielding this information, and in all such studies combined

Study	RR	95% CI	Significance
Williams and Horm, 1977	1.36	(1.13, 1.63)	p<0.001
Byers and Funch, 1982	1.08	(0.88, 1.32)	n.s.
Rosenberg et al., 1982	1.59	(1.32, 1.91)	p<0.001
Begg et al., 1983	1.19	(0.97, 1.45)	n.s.
Paganini-Hill and Ross, 1983	0.98	(0.66, 1.45)	n.s.
Webster et al., 1983	0.99	(0.80, 1.23)	n.s.
Hiatt and Bawol, 1984	1.05	(0.90, 1.22)	n.s.
Le et al., 1984	1.28	(1.00, 1.63)	p<0.05
Talamini et al., 1984	2.09	(1.48, 2.95)	p<0.001
La Vecchia et al., 1985	1.32	(0.97, 1.79)	n.s.
Katsouyami et al., 1986	0.80	(0.47, 1.37)	n.s.
Harvey et al., 1987	1.14	(0.97, 1.35)	n.s.
La Vecchia et al., 1987	1.59	(1.33, 1.90)	p<0.001
Schatzkin et al., 1987	1.60	(1.00, 2.50)	p<0.05
Willett et al., 1987	1.19	(1.00, 1.43)	p<0.05
Adami et al, 1988	1.03	(0.78, 1.34)	n.s.
Harris et al., 1988	0.98	(0.87, 1.12)	n.s.
Rohan and McMichael, 1988	1.07	(0.81, 1.41)	n.s.
Schatzkin, 1989b	0.90	(0.60, 1.20)	n.s.
Young, (aged <= 35): 1989 (aged > 35):	1.98 1.45	(1.43, 2.73) (1.03, 2.03)	p<0.001 p<0.05
All studies	1.20	(1.14, 1.26)	p<0.001

Significant heterogeneity among studies (chi-squared = 73.22, p<0.001)

Table 6.26: Dose-response trends in the log-odds ratios with increasing consumption, in litres of ethanol per week, in studies yielding sufficient information to estimate these, and in all such studies combined

Study	Trend	se(trend)	Significance
Byers and Funch, 1982	0.63	0.82	n.s.
Begg et al., 1983	1.95	0.93	p<0.05
Paganini-Hill and Ross, 1983	0.12	0.11	n.s.
Webster et al., 1983	0.26	0.40	n.s.
Hiatt and Bawol, 1983	1.03	0.29	p<0.001
Le et al., 1984	1.53	0.55	p<0.01
Talamini et al., 1984	4.13	0.89	p<0.001
La Vecchia et al., 1985	−0.18	0.40	n.s.
Harvey et al., 1987	1.37	0.48	p<0.01
La Vecchia et al., 1987	2.96	0.43	p<0.001
O'Connell et al., 1987	9.65	10.33	n.s.
Schatzkin et al., 1987	2.87	4.16	n.s.
Willett et al., 1987	3.31	0.61	p<0.001
Adami et al., 1988	−1.05	1.56	n.s.
Rohan and McMichael, 1988	3.41	1.50	p<0.05
Schatzkin et al., 1989	−11.89	5.37	p<0.05
Young, (age <= 35):	4.20	1.50	p<0.01
1989 (age > 35):	3.20	1.20	p<0.01
All studies	0.59	0.09	p<0.001

Significant heterogeneity among studies (chi-squared =150.86, p<0.001)

alcohol, effects of nutritional deficiencies associated with heavy drinking, and increased membrane permeability by other carcinogens due to the effect of alcohol.

There is no strong evidence of a beverage-specific effect. Indications of beverage-specific effects in individual papers can be seen on closer inspection to be a reflection of the most popular beverage in the area in which the study was conducted. Thus, for example, Talamini et al. (1984) in Italy, find a strong effect of wine consumption, whereas Rohan and McMichael (1988) in Australia find strong effects of beer and spirits.

In conclusion, while there is no consensus on a causal relationship, until the effect of alcohol consumption can be convincingly accounted for by adjustment for other variables, it must be treated as a predisposing factor.

6.6.4 Attributable risk

If we first consider attributable risk from any drinking at all, we have a relative risk of 1.20 from Table 6.25 and a prevalence of drinking among women in England and Wales of 92%. This yields an attributable risk of 16%. The annual mortality rate for female breast cancer in England and Wales is 523 per million (OPCS, 1989). So, elimination of all drinking would avoid 84 deaths per million women per year (i.e. 2,163 breast cancer deaths per year in total).

Considering the more achievable goal of reducing average consumption, the median alcohol consumption in England and Wales among women can be estimated as 32ml per week (see related document on bladder cancer). Using the trend estimate of 0.59 per litre per week from Table 26, suppose a reduction of 20ml per week. This is associated with a risk reduction of 1.2%, avoiding 6 deaths per million women per year (i.e. 155 deaths per year in England and Wales as a whole).

The fact that eliminating all drinking would seem to have a greater effect than the median consumption would suggest may be indicative of a quantitative difference between those who drink and those who do not, or of serious misreporting of the amount consumed. In any case, these results must be treated as tentative, being unadjusted for potential confounders, particularly dietary variables unmeasured or poorly measured in the various studies.

6.7 Alcohol and cancer of the pancreas

6.7.1 Published research

Thirty-four studies are reviewed in all. A qualitative summary is given in Table 6.27. Eight (Sundby, 1967; Schmidt and de Lint, 1972; Hakulinen, 1974; Monson and Lyon, 1975; Adelstein and White, 1976; Robinette et al., 1979; Schmidt and Popham, 1981; Prior, 1988) followed up cohorts of alcoholics. None found any significantly increased risk associated with alcoholism. Two (Dean et al., 1979; Jensen, 1979) followed up cohorts of brewery workers. Neither found any significant increase in risk in these workers.

Five (Blackwelder et al., 1980; Heuch et al., 1983; Hirayama, 1985; Kono et al., 1986; Hiatt et al., 1988b) followed up a cohort of (approximately) general population subjects. Only one (Heuch et al., 1983) found a signifi-

Table 6.27: Studies of alcohol and pancreatic cancer

Study	Design and Methods	Summary of qualitative results
Sundby, 1967	Cohort. 1,693 male alcoholics followed up for mortality.	No significant effect.
Ishii et al., 1973	Case-control. 475 cases, 122,261 historical controls. Drinkers compared to non-drinkers.	Increased risk (RR = 1.5) in drinkers, significance not stated.
Schmidt and de Lint, 1972	Cohort. 1,119 female alcoholics followed up for mortality.	No significant effect.
Wynder et al., 1973	Case-control. 142 cases, 307 age-, sex- and race-matched controls. Five consumption categories.	No significant effect.
Hakulinen et al., 1974	Cohort. Roughly 210,000 male alcohol-abusers followed up for incidence.	No significant effect.
Monson and Lyon, 1975	Cohort. 1,382 (1,139 male) alcoholics followed up for mortality.	No significant effect.
Adelstein and White, 1976	Cohort. 2,070 (1,595 male) alcoholics followed up for mortality.	No significant effect.
Williams and Horm, 1977	Case-control. 170 (113 male) cases, 5,574 (2,074 male) controls. Lifetime consumption in three categories.	No significant effect in either sex, adjusted for smoking.
Dean et al., 1979	Cohort. Male brewery workers (3–4000 in each of four five-year periods) followed up for mortality	No significant effect.
Jensen, 1979	Cohort. 14,313 male brewery workers followed up for incidence	No significant effect.
Robinette et al., 1979	Cohort. 4,401 male alcoholics and 4,401 controls followed up for mortality.	No significant effect.
Blackwelder et al., 1980	Cohort. Mortality in normal population (numbers unknown) studied in relation to mean consumption.	No significant effect.
Lin and Kessler, 1981	Case-control. 109 (67 male) cases, 109 age-, sex-, race- and marital status-matched controls.	Cases drank more wine than controls.
McMahon et al., 1981	Case-control. 367 (218 male) cases, 644 (307 male) controls. Three consumption categories.	No significant effect.

Table 6.27: (*Continued*)

Study	Design and Methods	Summary of qualitative results
Manousos et al., 1981	Case-control. 50 (32 male) cases, 206 (172 male) controls. Two consumption categories.	No significant effect.
Schmidt and Popham, 1981	Cohort. 9,889 male alcoholics followed up for mortality.	No significant effect.
Haines et al., 1982	Case-control. 116 (56 male) cases, 232 (112 male) controls. Three consumption categories.	No association observed. Data not shown.
Tuyns et al., 1982	Case-control. 42 cases, 1,976 controls. Drinkers compared to non-drinkers	No significant effect.
Durbec et al., 1983	Case-control. 69 (37 male) cases, 199 (100 male) controls. Intake in g/day. Beverage-specific analyses.	Higher consumption in cases ($p < 0.05$). RR = 1.24 for an increase of 10g/day.
Heuch et al., 1983	Cohort. 16,713 subjects followed up for incidence. Three consumption categories.	Significant trend of increasing risk with increasing consumption.
Kodama and Mori, 1983	Case-control. 76 case, 86 controls. Habitual daily use (yes/no).	No significant effect.
Wynder et al., 1983	Case-control. 275 (153 male) cases, 7,994 (5,469 male) controls. Five consumption categories.	No significant effect, but suggestion of increased risk in males in highest consumption group.
Gold et al., 1985	Case-control. 201 cases, 201 hospital, 201 community controls. Wine consumption in five categories.	Suggestion of negative association with consumption using community controls.
Hirayama, 1985	Cohort. Details not available.	No effect observed.
Kono et al., 1986	Cohort. 51,335 male Japanese doctors followed up for mortality. Four consumption categories.	No significant effect.
Mack et al., 1986	Case-control. 490 (282 male) cases, 490 matched controls. Four consumption categories. Beverage-specific analyses.	No significant effect.
Norell et al., 1986	Case-control. 99 (55 male) cases, 163 hospital, 138 population controls. Three consumption categories	No effect, or possible negative effect.
Raymond et al., 1987	Case-control. 88 cases, 336 controls. Beer and wine consumption (three categories).	Significant increase in risk with high beer consumption (RR = 2.9).

Table 6.27: (*Continued*)

Study	Design and Methods	Summary of qualitative results
Falk et al., 1988	Case-control. 363 (203 male) cases, 1,234 (890 male) controls. Varying categories for different beverages.	No significant effect.
Hiatt et al., 1988	Case-control within cohort study of 122,894 subjects. Alcohol consumption in drinks per day.	No significant effect.
Prior, 1988	Cohort. 1,110 (876 male) alcoholics followed up for incidence.	No significant effect.
Clavel et al., 1989	Case-control. 161 (98 male) cases, 268 (161 male) hospital controls. Five consumption categories.	No significant effect.
Cuzick and Babiker, 1989	Case-control. 216 (123 male) cases, 279 (150 male) hospital and general practice controls. Categories vary by beverage.	Significant increase in risk with high beer intake (RR = 3.2).
Olsen et al., 1989	Case-control. 212 male cases, 220 male population controls. Four consumption categories. Beverage-specific analyses.	Suggestion of increased risk with 4 or more drinks per day (RR = 2.7) compared to non-drinkers.

cant positive effect of alcohol consumption on risk of pancreatic cancer, and in this study the results are difficult to interpret due to selection in the formation of the cohort and differing results depending on whether the cases were histologically confirmed (IARC, 1988).

The remaining nineteen studies are case-control studies (see Table 6.27). Of these, four (Durbec et al., 1983; Raymond et al., 1987; Cuzick and Babiker, 1989; Olsen et al., 1989) find significant, or almost significant, increases in risk associated with consumption of alcohol of one form or another. Two in particular (Raymond et al., 1987; Cuzick and Babiker, 1989) find an increased risk in association with high beer consumption.

The large number of studies indicate that the question has been repeatedly researched and that a quantitative overview of the case-control studies should be informative. In the following overviews, only case-control studies are used since only one cohort study provided data in a suitable form.

6.7.2 Partial quantitative overview

Alcohol as a binary risk factor. Studies assessing (or reporting data in such a way as to enable assessment of) whether drinkers have a higher risk of

Table 6.28: Relative risks of pancreatic cancer for drinkers compared to non-drinkers

Study	RR	(95% CI)	Significance
Wynder et al., 1973	1.34	(0.87, 2.06)	n.s.
Williams and Horm, 1977	1.47	(1.05, 2.04)	p<0.05
McMahon et al., 1981	1.00	(0.68, 1.46)	n.s.
Tuyns et al., 1982	1.07	(0.08, 13.53)	n.s.
Wynder et al., 1983	1.07	(0.80, 1.43)	n.s.
Gold et al., 1985	0.55	(0.25, 1.19)	n.s.
Mack et al., 1986	0.82	(0.58, 1.15)	n.s.
Falk et al., 1988	1.31	(0.85, 2.01)	n.s.
Clavel et al., 1989	0.72	(0.45, 1.14)	n.s.
Cuzick and Babiker, 1989	1.12	(0.60, 2.07)	n.s.
Olsen et al., 1989	0.70	(0.44, 1.10)	n.s.
All studies	1.03	(0.90, 1.17)	n.s.

Significant heterogeneity among studies, $p < 0.05$

pancreatic cancer than non-drinkers are shown in Table 6.28, with the relative risk for drinkers compared to non-drinkers in each study. The pooled estimate from all studies combined is given at the bottom of the table. Overall, there appears to be no effect, although the significant heterogeneity among studies suggests caution in interpreting this.

Dose-response. For those studies reporting sufficient information to estimate dose-response trends, results are shown in Table 6.29, with the associated combined estimate. The combined estimate of 0.0018 is equiv-

Table 6.29: Trends in the log-odds ratio for pancreatic cancer with increasing alcohol consumption in ml/day

Study	Trend	Standard Error	Significance
Wynder et al., 1973	0.0033	0.0023	n.s.
Durbec et al., 1983	0.0269	0.0106	p<0.05
Kodama and Mori, 1983	−0.0101	0.0065	n.s.
Wynder et al., 1983	0.0063	0.0044	n.s.
Mack et al., 1985	0.0021	0.0019	n.s.
Norell et al., 1986	−0.0615	0.0214	p<0.01
Falk et al., 1988	−0.0021	0.0025	n.s.
Clavell et al., 1989 (males)	−0.0056	0.0050	n.s.
Clavell et al., 1989 (females)	−0.0075	0.0073	n.s.
Cuzick and Babiker, 1989	0.0122	0.0090	n.s.
Olsen et al., 1989	0.0167	0.0055	p<0.01
All studies	0.0018	0.0011	n.s.

Significant heterogeneity among studies, $p < 0.001$

alent to a relative risk of 1.02 in association with an increased consumption of 10.5ml of ethanol per day (e.g. half a pint of beer) or of 1.21 with an increased consumption of 105ml of ethanol (e.g. five pints of beer). Thus the risk, if a risk exists, is small. In any case, the combined trend is not significantly different from zero. There is significant heterogeneity from study to study however, so there may in fact be a larger or a negative effect.

6.7.3 Is there a biological link?

While alcohol is known to affect pancreatic function (see for example Potter et al., 1982), there is no consensus that alcohol affects the pancreas as a carcinogen. The overall negative results of Tables 6.24 and 6.25, together with the lack of an effect of alcoholism, bear out this conclusion. While Cuzick and Babiker (1989) and Raymond et al. (1987) found effects of beer consumption in particular, these are not borne out by studies on cohorts of brewery workers, who have higher beer consumption than the general population, so they may be chance results. Their apparent dependence on particular cut-off points is another reason to view them with caution. In all, it appears that there is no biological effect of alcohol on pancreatic cancer risk.

6.7.4 Attributable risk

The overall estimate of relative risk associated with any drinking at all is 1.03. The prevalence of drinking in England and Wales is estimated as 95% in men and 92% in women (Goddard and Ikin, 1989). These give an attributable risk of 3% in both men and women. Mortality from cancer of the pancreas is 118 per million per year in men and 116 per million per year in women (OPCS, 1989). A decrease of 3% would therefore change these rates to 114 for men and 113 for women, saving a total of 175 lives per year in England and Wales, by eliminating all drinking. Of course, this is not feasible and in any case, the non-significance of the effect indicates that we could not confidently expect even this benefit.

Consider now the effect of simply a reduction in average daily consumption. Using Table 2.12 of Goddard and Ikin (1989), we estimate median daily consumptions of 21ml in men and 5ml in women. If these were halved, the combined estimate of Table 6.29 would give risk reductions of 2% in men and 0.5% in women, thus reducing the rates to 116 per million per year for men and 115 for women, saving a total of 75 lives per year. Once again, the non-significance of the result casts doubt on even this benefit.

Although the studies displayed significant heterogeneity, the overall negative results of the studies on alcoholics suggest that these very small risk estimates are approximately correct.

6.8 Alcohol and bladder cancer

6.8.1 Published research

Studies assessing alcohol and bladder cancer risk are shown in Table 6.30, with a brief qualitative summary of the results of each study. Of the fifteen studies available, eight (Wynder et al., 1963; Dunham et al., 1968; Pell and D'Alonzo, 1973; Morgan and Jain, 1974; Hakulinen et al., 1974; Monson and Lyon, 1975; Thomas et al., 1983; Brownsen et al., 1987) found no significant effect of alcohol on bladder cancer risk, whether crude or adjusted. Two (Williams and Horm, 1977; Mommsen et al., 1982) found a significant increase in risk associated with alcohol when analysed unadjusted, but which disappears when adjusted for tobacco habit. A further two (Claude et al., 1986; Kaisary et al., 1987) found an increased risk associated with alcohol only among smokers. Hirayama (1979) found an increased risk (significance not stated) associated with alcohol consumption among smokers but did not quote the results for non-smokers. One study (Risch et al., 1988) found a significant trend of increasing risk with alcohol consumption after adjustment for smoking, among females. Slattery et al. (1988) found a borderline significant increase in risk with alcohol use and reported that this was still present when adjusted for smoking, although the adjusted result was not explicitly quoted.

The cohort studies are of limited use here. Hirayama (1979) did not report significance, standard errors or tabulated data, and the other cohort studies (Pell and D'Alonzo, 1973; Hakulinen et al., 1974; Monson and Lyon, 1975) compared bladder cancer incidence in alcoholic patients with the incidence in non-alcoholics, and so did not directly assess consumption.

Four studies assessed risk by type of beverage (Williams and Horm, 1977; Thomas et al., 1983; Claude et al., 1986; Risch et al., 1988).

6.8.2 Partial quantitative overview

Dose response. Four studies reported on their data in sufficient detail to assess a trend in risk with increasing alcohol consumption. These are shown in Table 6.31, with individual and combined estimates of trend. The overall effect in females is significant ($p < 0.05$), indicating an increase in risk of 2.04 per litre of ethanol per week (i.e., a 2% increase per 10ml per week), with 95% confidence interval (1.03, 1.39). There is no significant effect among males, and the results for males vary significantly from study to study ($p < 0.01$), rendering the combined estimate difficult to interpret. Similarly the results for males differ significantly from those for females ($p < 0.01$).

Drinking as a binary risk factor. Several studies reported data on drinking as a dichotomous factor (i.e. comparing risk in drinkers with risk in non-drinkers). These studies are shown in Table 6.32, with odds-ratio relative risk estimates, in individual studies and in all studies combined. These were also combined by Woolf's method. In males alone and in males and females

Table 6.30: Design and brief summaries of results of studies of bladder cancer and alcohol

Study, year	Design	Subjects	Alcohol classification	Qualitative results*
Wynder et al., 1963	Case-control	Males, 200 cases 200 ctrls	Drinks per day, 7 classes	No significant effect
Dunham et al., 1968	Case-control	Males and females, 493 cases 527 ctrls	Ounces per week, 2 classes	No significant effect (data not shown)
Pell and D'Alonzo, 1973	Cohort	Numbers not known	Alcoholic/ non-alcoholic	No significant effect
Morgan and Jain, 1974	Case-control	Both sexes, 229 cases 231 ctrls	Drink/ do not drink	No significant effect
Hakulinen et al., 1974	Cohort	Males, 4,370 subjects	Alcoholic/ non-alcoholic	No significant effect
Monson and Lyon, 1975	Cohort	Males, 894 subjects	Alcoholic/ non-alcoholic	No significant effect
Williams and Horm, 1977	Case-control	Both sexes, 306 cases 5,566 ctrls	Not clear from text	Significant effect annulled by adjusting for smoking
Hirayama, 1979	Cohort	Not known	At least 1 drink per day	Elevated relative risk for drinkers, significance not reported
Mommsen et al., 1982	Case-control	Males, 165 cases 165 ctrls	Drink/ do not drink	Almost significant effect annulled by adjusting for smoking.
Thomas et al.,	Case-control	Both sexes, 2,982 cases, 5,782 ctrls	Drinks per week, 7 classes	No significant effect
Claude et al., 1986	Case-control	Both sexes, 431 cases, 431 ctrls	Litres per day of beverage	Significant effect among smokers
Brownson et al., 1987	Case-control	Males, 823 cases, 2,469 ctrls	Drinks per day, 3 classes	No significant effect
Kaisary et al., 1987	Case-control	Both sexes, 99 cases, 110 ctrls	Drink/ do not drink	Significant effect among smokers
Risch et al., 1988	Case-control	Both sexes, 826 cases, 792 ctrls	Trends in ethanol	Significant trend in females
Slattery et al., 1988	Case-control	Males, 332 cases, 686 ctrls	Drink/ do not drink	Almost significant effect

*Unless otherwise stated, significant effects refer to positive associations.

Table 6.31: Combined estimates of trend in log odds ratio risk estimate per litre of ethanol per week

Study, year	Number of cases	Trend	S.E. (trend)
(a) Males			
Wynder et al., 1963	200	0.1260	0.2362
Thomas et al., 1983	2,226	0.1980	0.0981
Brownson et al., 1987	607	0.2929	0.4493
Risch et al., 1988	Not given	−0.2176	0.1110
(b) Females			
Thomas et al., 1983	756	0.5492	0.3659
Risch et al., 1988	Not given	2.0370	1.0393
Males, combined*		0.0318	0.0693
Females, combined[+]		0.7133	0.3451
All studies, both sexes[o]		0.0582	0.0679

*Significant heterogeneity among studies, $p < 0.01$
[+]Trend significant, $p < 0.05$
[o]Significant heterogeneity between male and female results, $p < 0.01$

Table 6.32: Combination of relative risks for bladder cancer for drinking compared to not drinking

Study, year	Number of cases	OR	(95% CI)	Significance
(a) Males				
Williams and Horm, 1977	229	1.16	(0.87, 1.54)	n.s.
Mommsen et al., 1982	165	2.46	(0.92, 6.56)	n.s.
Thomas et al., 1983	2,256	1.01	(0.90, 1.13)	n.s.
Brownsen et al., 1987	823	1.19	(0.98, 1.44)	n.s.
Slattery et al., 1988	332	1.28	(0.97, 1.69)	n.s.
(b) Females				
Williams and Horm, 1987	77	0.88	(0.48, 1.62)	n.s.
Thomas et al., 1983	756	1.04	(0.86, 1.25)	n.s.
Male studies combined*	3,775	1.09	(0.99, 1.18)	$0.1 > p > 0.05$
Female studies combined	833	1.03	(0.86, 1.23)	n.s.
All studies combined	4,608	1.07	(0.99, 1.16)	$0.1 > p > 0.05$

*Significant heterogeneity among studies.

combined, the increased risk associated with drinking approached statistical significance $(0.1 > p > 0.05)$, indicating an 8% increase in risk associated with drinking in males, although the effect of drinking in males was hetero-geneous among studies $(p < 0.05)$, indicating that this combined estimate is of questionable value.

6.8.3 Is there a biological relationship?

The results of the above are consistent with a small increase in risk of bladder cancer associated with alcohol consumption, but, before discussing the biological implications, certain caveats should be made clear. First, to perform the quantitative overview, the data had to be available in the publication (except in the case of Risch et al. (1988), where only the trends were explicitly reported, adjusted for smoking), and was invariably not cross-tabulated with smoking habit (with the exception of Slattery's paper, which unfortunately did not present data for males and females separately). Since smoking is shown to account for the relationship between alcohol and risk in two of the five studies used in Table 6.3 (Williams and Horm, 1977; Mommsen et al., 1982), these estimates are probably anticonservative, i.e. the association of alcohol with risk is actually smaller than that estimated. Also, there is evidence (Claude et al., 1986; Kaisary et al., 1988) that the effect of drinking is only observed in smokers. It should also be noted that, although not suitable for numerical combination, the results of the cohort studies do not indicate any substantial excess risk among alcoholics.

If there can be said to be a consensus, it is that the effect of alcohol on bladder cancer risk is minimal, if it exists at all (International Agency for Research on Cancer, 1988). Possible mechanisms for such a relationship are:

1. Irritation of the site by contact with alcohol.
2. Carcinogenic effects of non-alcohol impurities in beverages (e.g. nitros-amines in some beverages).
3. Nutritional deficiencies associated with problem drinking.
4. Alcohol may act as a solvent for other carcinogens, hence making them more easily absorbed.
5. Alcohol consumption is confounded with smoking, but may also be confounded with unmeasured effects of smoking residual to classification (e.g. to the difference between 20 cigarettes per day and 40 per day in a study where both are classified as '20+').

These possible mechanisms are discussed in more detail by Thomas et al. (1983) and Claude et al. (1986). Since no effect of high consumption consistent across many studies was observed (and no effect of alcoholism in the cohort studies), (1) would seem unlikely. If (2) were true, the effect would be beverage-specific.

There is no strong indication of a beverage-specific effect from the studies reporting on beer, wine and spirit drinking separately (Williams and

Horm, 1977; Thomas et al., 1983; Claude et al., 1986; Risch et al., 1988). Unfortunately, the beverage-specific results are not reported in a manner facilitating their numerical combination. The fact that the cohort studies specifically studying alcoholics have largely negative results is evidence against (3). Possibilities (4) and (5) are plausible, in view of the findings of Claude et al. (1986) and Kaisary et al. (1987) that the increase in risk associated with drinking is confined to smokers. Thus it may be that alcohol-drinking, while having no universal effect on bladder cancer risk, may exacerbate or seem to exacerbate the effect of smoking on risk.

6.8.4 Attributable risk and mortality

The combined estimates for males and females in Table 6.31 can be used to estimate risks for different levels of consumption. The mortality rates per 100,000 in 1987 were 11.9 for males and 5.5 for females (Office of Population Censuses and Surveys, 1989). Median alcohol consumption was approximately 148ml per week (13 units) for men and 32ml (3 units) for women, calculated from Table 2.12 in Goddard and Ikin (1989). A shift of the former down to say 50ml per week would incur a 0.4% reduction in risk, leaving the figure of 11.9 deaths per 100,000 per year virtually unchanged. In females, a reduction to say 10ml weekly would incur a 2% reduction in risk, reducing the death rate to 5.4 per 100,000, saving between 20 and 30 lives.

Using the combined estimates of Table 6.32, we obtain attributable risks of 8% in males and 3% in females; that is, by eliminating drinking altogether, we would reduce incidence (and presumably mortality) by 8% in males and 3% in females, thus bringing the male death rate down to 10.9 and the female to 5.3. However, complete elimination of drinking is not a feasible strategy.

Since these figures are based on estimates unadjusted for smoking, they are probably overestimates of the effect of alcohol, and should be regarded as the maximum possible hypothetical benefits. Further, only the trend estimate for females is unequivocally significantly different from no effect. Thus, this overview does not provide evidence for believing otherwise than that the effect of alcohol on bladder cancer risk is minimal, or that changing alcohol consumption is likely to save more than a small percentage of lives which would otherwise have been lost.

6.9 Alcohol and risk of liver cancer

6.9.1 Published research

Published studies are shown in Table 6.33. Twenty-one studies are reviewed, of which eleven (Adelstein and White, 1976; Dean et al., 1979; Hakulinen, 1974; Jensen, 1980; Kono et al., 1986; Monson and Lyon, 1975; Prior, 1988; Robinette et al., 1979; Schmidt and Popham, 1981; Shibata,

Table 6.33: Design and brief summaries of results of studies of cancer of the liver reviewed

Study	Design	Qualitative results
Schwartz, 1962	Case-control. 61 cases, 61 controls. Consumption per day.	No significant differences in quantity, type or age of starting to drink, but cases drank more than controls. No adjustment for smoking.
Sundby, 1967*	Cohort. Alcoholics followed up for death from liver cancer. 1,693 males.	Non-significantly increased risk associated with alcoholism (RR = 2.0).
Hakulinen, 1974	Cohort. 210,000 male alcohol-abusers followed up for liver cancer incidence.	Significant increase in risk among alcohol-misusers. RR = 1.49.
Monson and Lyon, 1975	Cohort. 1,382 alcoholics followed up for mortality.	No significant association of alcoholism with risk.
Adelstein and White, 1976	Cohort. 2,070 (1,595 male) alcoholics followed up for mortality.	Significantly increased risk for male alcoholics. RR = 6.4.
Williams and Horm, 1977	Case-control. 28 cases (18 male), 4,948 (1,770 male) controls with other malignancies. Lifetime consumption.	After adjustment for smoking, non-significant increases in risk with consumption.
Dean et al., 1979	Cohort. Male brewery workers (3–4000 in each of four five-year periods) followed up for mortality.	No significant effect. RR = 1.3.
Robinette et al., 1979	Cohort. 4,401 alcoholics and 4,401 controls followed up for mortality.	No significant association of risk with alcoholism.
Infante et al., 1980	Case-control. 35 cases (31 male) and 433 controls (207 male. Daily and lifelong consumption.	Consumption of cases twice as high as that of controls.
Jensen, 1980	Cohort. 14,313 brewery workers followed up for incidence and mortality.	Significantly increased risk among beer production workers (RR = 1.5).
Schmidt and Popham, 1981	Cohort. 9,889 male alcoholics followed up for mortality.	Non-significantly increased risk with alcoholism (RR = 2.0).
Bulatao-Jayme et al., 1982	Case-control. 90 cases, 90 controls. Light and heavy consumption categories, compared adjusted for aflatoxin intakes.	Significant effect of consumption on risk (RR = 3.8). Significance remained when adjusted for aflatoxins.
Lam et al., 1982	Case-control. 107 cases, 107 age- and sex-matched controls.	No significant effect (no quantitative details given).
Stemhagen et al., 1983	Case-control. 265 (178 male) cases, 530 age-, sex-, race- and residence-matched controls. Annual consumption.	Significant trend of increasing risk with consumption in females.

Table 6.33: (*Continued*)

Study	Design	Qualitative results
Yu et al., 1983	Case-control. 78 cases (50 male), 78 age-, sex-, race- and residence-matched controls. Daily consumption.	Significant increase in risk with high consumption. Significance remains when adjusted for smoking.
Hardell et al., 1984	Case-control. 83 dead male cases and 199 dead male controls. Approximate weekly consumption.	Significant increase in risk among those with high consumption, with or without adjustment for smoking.
Austin et al., 1986	Case-control. 86 cases (60 male), 161 controls. Broad consumption categories.	Significant increasing trend in risk with consumption, adjusted for smoking.
Kono et al., 1986	Cohort. 5,135 males classified by consumption followed up for mortality.	Significant increased risk associated with high consumption.
Shibata et al. 1986	Cohort. 1,316 Japanese males, classified by sake and shochu drinking, followed up for mortality.	Significant increase in risk with high shochu consumption (RR = 7.5).
Trichopoulos et al., 1987	Case-control. 173 cases, 400 controls.	No significant association of consumption with risk.
Prior, 1988	Cohort. 1,110 alcoholics followed up for incidence. In cubic cm/day (3 categories).	Significantly elevated risk among male alcoholics. RR – 38.1.

1986; Sundby, 1967) are cohort studies and ten (Austin et al., 1986; Bulatao-Jayme et al., 1982; Hardell et al., 1984; Infante et al., 1980; Lam et al., 1982; Schwartz et al., 1962; Stemhagen et al., 1983; Trichopoulos et al., 1987; Williams and Horm, 1977; Yu et al., 1983) are case-control studies. The overall impression is that the subject has been adequately researched, that there is an increased risk in association with alcohol-drinking (since the effects are virtually all in a positive direction whether significant or not), and that the effect of drinking is not attributable to smoking.

6.9.2 Partial quantitative overview

Dose-response. Four studies gave sufficient information for a quantitative trend overview (Table 6.34). The overall effect is significant, with a logistic regression coefficient of 0.0066 per ml of ethanol per day. This corresponds to a relative risk of 1.14 associated with an increased consumption of one pint of beer per day. No significant heterogeneity among studies was observed. The trend is significant in each study, including the one with adjustment for smoking (Yu et al., 1983).

Drinking as a binary risk factor. Six studies gave sufficient information to assess the effect of drinking compared with not drinking (Table 6.35). The overall estimate of relative risk for drinkers compared to non-drinkers was

Table 6.34: Trends in the log-odds ratio relative risk estimate for liver cancer with alcohol consumption in ml/day of ethanol

Study	Trend	SE	Significance
Stemhagen et al., 1983	0.0064	0.0022	p<0.01
Yu et al., 1983	0.0151	0.0059	p<0.05
Kono et al. 1986	0.0087	0.0044	p<0.05
Trichopoulos et al., 1987	0.0050	0.0023	p<0.05
All studies	0.0066	0.0014	p<0.001

No significant heterogeneity among studies.

1.56 (p<0.001). Note that all studies show an effect in the same direction. There was no significant heterogeneity among studies.

6.9.3 Is there a biological relationship?

The overall indications are that there is a causal relationship between alcohol-drinking and liver cancer (International Agency for Research on Cancer, 1988). This may be by direct damage to the liver or by association with other risk factors. There is some evidence that alcohol drinking enhances the predisposing effect of the Hepatitis B virus (Oshima et al., 1984).

6.9.4 Attributable risk

The combined relative risk estimate for any drinking at all was 1.56. With Goddard and Ikin's (1989) male and female prevalence figures of 95% and 92% respectively, we obtain attributable risks of 35% for men and 34% for women. In England and Wales in 1987, there were 726 deaths from liver cancer among males and 526 among women. Eliminating all drinking would therefore avoid 254 deaths among men and 179 deaths among women.

Taking the more modest aim of halving consumption, the combined trend was 0.0066 per ml of ethanol per day. Median consumption in

Table 6.35: Relative risks of liver cancer for drinkers compared to non-drinkers

Study	RR	95% CI	Significance
Williams and Horm, 1977	1.66	(0.77, 3.56)	n.s.
Stemhagen et al., 1983	1.39	(0.92, 2.11)	n.s.
Hardell et al., 1984	2.65	(1.13, 6.20)	p<0.05
Austin et al., 1986	1.64	(0.89, 3.02)	n.s.
Kono et al., 1986	1.75	(0.89, 3.42)	n.s.
Shibata et al., 1986	1.19	(0.60, 2.36)	n.s.
All studies	1.56	(1.21, 2.00)	p<0.001

No significant heterogeneity among studies.

England and Wales is roughly 21ml per day for men and 5ml per day for women (Goddard and Ikin, 1989). Halving these figures would lead to risk reductions of 7% in men and 2% in women, avoiding 51 male deaths and 11 female.

6.10 Conclusion

The International Agency for Research on Cancer's (1988) monograph concluded that alcohol is causally related to cancers of the oral cavity, pharynx, larynx, oesophagus and liver. This work is in agreement with that conclusion and suggests that breast cancer should probably be added to the list of cancers caused by alcohol-drinking. The size, however, of the effect of alcohol-drinking on breast cancer risk is heterogeneous between studies and indicates that further work is needed. It may well be that there is an underlying effect of alcohol on breast cancer risk but that an unobserved confounding variable, probably dietary, is varying significantly among the populations in which the various studies are carried out. Carefully-conducted prospective studies are necessary to achieve a consensus on the effect of alcohol consumption on risk of breast cancer.

It is also possible that drinking alcohol increases the risks of cancers of the large bowel and possibly the stomach. Again, however, effects vary significantly from study to study.

Approximate quantitative overviews suggest that alcohol consumption as a whole is responsible for about 2500 deaths per year in England and Wales from cancers of the mouth, pharynx, larynx, oesophagus and liver. If the results on breast cancer and colorectal cancer are correct, the number of cancer deaths per year attributable to alcohol would be about 7500.

References

Adami, H.O., Lind, E., Bergström, R. and Meirik, O. (1988) Cigarette smoking, alcohol consumption and risk of breast cancer in young women, *British Journal of Cancer* 58: 832–7.

Adelstein, A. and White, G. (1976) Alcoholism and mortality, *Population Trends* 6: 7–13.

Austin, H., Delzell, E., Grufferman, S., Levine, R., Morrison, A.S., Stolley, P.D. and Cole, P. (1986) A case-control study of hepatocellular carcinoma and the hepatitis B virus, cigarette smoking and alcohol consumption, *Cancer Research* 46: 962–6.

Begg, C.B., Walker, A.M., Wessen, B. and Zelen, M. (1983) Alcohol consumption and breast cancer, *Lancet* i: 293–4.

Bjelke, E. (1973) Epidemiologic studies of cancer of the stomach, colon and rectum with special emphasis on the role of diet, Doctoral Thesis, University of Minnesota.

Blackwelder, W.C., Yano, K., Rhoads, G.G., Kagan, A., Gordon, T. and Palsch, Y. (1980) Alcohol and mortality: the Honolulu Heart Study, *American Journal of Cancer* 68: 164–9.

Blot, W.J., McLaughlin, J.K., Winn, D.M., Austin, D.F., Greenberg, R.S., Preston-Martin, S., Bernstein, L., Schoenberg, J.B., Stemhagen, J.B. and Fraumeni, J.F. (1988) Smoking and drinking in relation to oral and pharyngeal cancer, *Cancer Research* 48: 3282–7.

Bradshaw, E. and Schonland, M. (1969) Oesophageal and lung cancers in Natal African males in relation to certain socioeconomic factors. An analysis of 484 interviews, *British Journal of Cancer* 23: 275–84.

Bradshaw, E. and Schonland, M. (1974) Smoking, drinking and oesophageal cancer in African males of Johannesburg, South Africa, *British Journal of Cancer* 30: 157–63.

Breslow, N.E. and Day, N.E. (1980) *Statistical Methods in Cancer Research, I. The Analysis of Case-control Studies*, Lyon: IARC.

Bross, I.D.J. and Coombs, J. (1976) Early onset of oral cancer among women who drink and smoke, *Oncology* 33: 136–9.

Brown L.M., Blot W.J., Schuman S.H., Smith V.M., Ershaw A.G., Marks R.D. and Fraumeni J.F. (1988) Environmental factors and high risk of esophageal cancer among men in coastal South Carolina, *Journal of the National Cancer Institute* 80: 1620–5.

Brown, L.M., Mason, T.J., Pickle, L.W. Stewart, P.A., Buffler, P.A., Burau, K., Ziegler, R.G. and Fraumeni, J.F. (1988) Occupational risk factors for laryngeal cancer on the Texas Gulf coast. *Cancer Research* 48: 1960–4.

Brownsen, R.C., Chang, J.C. and Davis, J.R. (1987) Occupation, smoking and alcohol in the epidemiology of bladder cancer, *American Journal of Public Health* 77: 1298–300.

Brugere, J., Guenel, P., Leclerc, A. and Rodriguez, J. (1986) Differential effects of tobacco and alcohol in cancer of the larynx, pharynx and mouth, *Cancer* 57: 391–5.

Bulatao-Jayme, J., Almero, E.M., Castro Ma, C.A., Jardeleza Ma, T.R. and Salamat, L.A. (1982) A case-control dietary study of primary liver cancer risk from aflatoxin exposure, *International Journal of Epidemiology* 11: 112–119.

Burch, J.D., Howe, G.R., Miller, A.B. and Smemciw, R. (1981) Tobacco, alcohol, asbestos and nickel in the etiology of cancer of the larynx: a case-control study. *Journal of the National Cancer Institute* 67: 1219–24.

Byers, T. and Funch, D.P. (1982) Alcohol and breast cancer, *Lancet* i: 799–800.

Claude, J., Kunze, E., Frentzel-Beyme, R., Paczkowski, K., Schneider, J. and Schubert, H. (1986) Life-style and occupational risk factors in cancer of the lower urinary tract, *American Journal of Epidemiology* 124: 578–89.

Cuzick, J. and Babiker, A.G. (1989) Pancreatic cancer, alcohol, diabetes mellitus and gall-bladder disease, *International Journal of Cancer* 43: 415–21.

Day, N.E., Munoz, N. and Ghadirian, P. (1982) Epidemiology of esophageal cancer: a review, in Correa, P. and Haenzsel, W. (eds) *Epidemiology of cancer of the digestive tract*, The Hague: Martinus Nijhoff.

Dean, G., MacLennan, R., McLoughlin, H. and Shelley, E. (1979) Causes of death of blue-collar workers at a Dublin brewery, 1954–73, *British Journal of Cancer* 40: 581–9.

De Jong, U.W., Breslow, N., Goh Ewe Hong, J., Sridharan, M. and Shamugaratnam, K. (1974) Aetiological factors in oesophageal cancer in Singapore Chinese, *International Journal of Cancer* 13: 291–303.

De Stefani, E., Correa, P., Oreggia, F., Leira, J., Rivero, S., Fernandez, G., Deneo-Pellegrini, H., Zavala, D. and Fonthani, E. (1987) Risk factors for laryngeal cancer, *Cancer* 60: 3087–91.

Dunham, L.J., Rabson, A.S., Stewart, H.L., Frank, A.S. and Young, J.L. (1968) Rates, interview and pathology study of cancer of the urinary bladder in New Orleans, Louisiana, *Journal of the National Cancer Institute* 41: 683–709.

Duffy, S.W., Rohan, T.E. and Day, N.E. (1989) Misclassification in more than one factor in a case-control study: a combination of Mantel-Haenszel and maximum likelihood approaches, *Statistics in Medicine* 8: 1529–36.

Durbec, J.P., Chevillotte, G., Bidart, J.M., Berthezene, P. and Sarles, H. (1983) Diet, alcohol, tobacco and risk of cancer of the pancreas: a case-control study, *British Journal of Cancer* 47: 463–70.

Elwood, J.M., Pearson, J.C.G., Skippen, D.H. and Jackson, S.M. (1984) Alcohol, smoking, social and occupational factors in the aetiology of cancer of the oral cavity, pharynx and larynx, *International Journal of Cancer* 34: 603–12.

Falk, R.T., Pickle, L.W., Forthan, E.T., Correa, P. and Fraumeni, J.F. (1988) Life-style risk factors for pancreatic cancer in Louisiana: a case-control study, *American Journal of Epidemiology* 128: 324–36.

Feldman, J.G., Hazam, M., Nagarajam, M. and Kissin, B. (1975) A case-control investigation of alcohol, tobacco and diet in head and neck cancer, *Preventive Medicine* 4: 444–63.

Franco, E.L., Kowalski, L.P., Oliveira, B.V., Curado, M.P., Pereira, R.N., Silva, M.E., Fara, A.S. and Torloni, H. (1989) Risk factors for oral cancer in Brazil: a case-control study, *International Journal of Cancer* 43: 992–1000.

Gold, E.B., Gordis, L., Diener, M.D., Seltzer, R., Boitnott, J.K., Bynum, T.E. and Hutcheon, D.F. (1985) Diet and other risk factors for cancer of the pancreas, *Cancer* 55: 460–7.

Goddard, E. and Ikin, C. (1989) *Drinking in England and Wales in 1987*, London: Her Majesty's Stationery Office.

Gordon, T. and Kannel, W.B. (1984) Drinking and mortality: the Framingham study, *American Journal of Epidemiology* 120: 97–107.

Graham, S., Dayal, H., Rohrer, T., Swanson, M., Sultz, H., Shedd, D. and Fischman, D. (1977) Dentition, diet, tobacco and alcohol in the epidemiology of oral cancer, *Journal of the National Cancer Institute* 59: 1611–1618.

Graham, S., Schotz, W. and Martino, P. (1972) Alimentary factors in the epidemiology of gastric cancer, *Cancer* 30: 927–38.

Guenel, P., Chastang, J.F., Luce, D., Leclerc, A. and Brugere, J. (1988) A study of the interaction of alcohol-drinking and tobacco-smoking among French cases of laryngeal cancer, *Journal of Epidemiology and Community Health* 42: 350–4.

Haenszel, W., Kurihara, M., Segi, M. and Lee, R.K.C. (1972) Stomach cancer among Japanese in Hawaii, *Journal of the National Cancer Institute* 49: 969–988.

Haines, A.P., Moss, A.R., Whittemore, A. and Quivey, J. (1982) A case-control study of pancreatic carcinoma, *Journal of Cancer Research and Clinical Oncology* 103: 93–7.

Hakulinen, T., Lehtimaki, L., Lehtonen, M., Teppo, L. (1974) Cancer morbidity among two male cohorts with increased alcohol consumption in Finland, *Journal of the National Cancer Institute* 52: 1711–14.

Hardell, L., Bengtsson, N.O., Jonsson, U., Eriksson, S. and Larsson, L.G. (1984) Aetiological aspects on primary liver cancer with special regard to alcohol, organic solvents and acute intermittent porphyria – an epidemiological investigation, *British Journal of Cancer* 50: 389–97.

Harris, R.E. and Wynder, E.L. (1988) Breast cancer and alcohol consumption: a study in weak associations, *Journal of the American Medical Association* 259: 2867–71.

Harvey, E.B., Schairer, C., Brinton, L.A., Hoover, R.N. and Fraumeni, J.F. (1987) Alcohol consumption and breast cancer, *Journal of the National Cancer Institute* 78: 657–61.

Hebert, J.R. and Kabat, G.C. (1989) Menthol cigarette-smoking and oesophageal cancer, *International Journal of Epidemiology* 18: 37–44.

Herity, B., Moriarty, M., Daly, L., Dunn, J. and Bourke, G.J. (1982) The role of tobacco and alcohol in the aetiology of lung and larynx cancer, *British Journal of Cancer* 46: 961–4.

Heuch, I., Kvåle, G., Jacobsen, B.K. and Bjelke, E. (1983) Use of alcohol, tobacco and coffee and risk of pancreatic cancer, *British Journal of Cancer* 48: 637–43.

Hiatt, R.A. and Bawol, R.D. (1984) Alcoholic beverage consumption and breast cancer incidence, *American Journal of Epidemiology* 120: 676–83.

Hiatt, R.A., Klatsky, A.L. and Armstrong, M.A. (1988a) Alcohol consumption and the risk of breast cancer in a pre-paid health plan, *Cancer Research* 48: 2284–7.

Hiatt, R.A., Klatsky, A.L. and Armstrong, M.A. (1988b) Pancreatic cancer, blood glucose and beverage consumption, *International Journal of Cancer* 41: 794–7.

Higginson, J. (1966) Etiological factors in gastrointestinal cancer in man, *Journal of the National Cancer Institute* 37: 527–45.

Hinds, M.W., Thomas, D.B. and O'Reilly, H.P. (1979) Asbestos, dental X-rays, tobacco and alcohol in the epidemiology of laryngeal cancer, *Cancer* 44: 1114–20.

Hirayama, T. (1966) An epidemiological study of oral and pharyngeal cancer in Central and South-East Asia, *Bulletin of the World Health Organisation* 34: 41–9.

Hirayama, T. (1979) Diet and Cancer, *Nutrition and Cancer* 1: 67–81.

Hirayama, T. (1985) A cohort study on cancer in Japan, in Blot, W.J., Hirayama, T. and Hoel, D.G. (eds) *Statistical methods for cancer epidemiology*, Hiroshima: Radiation Effects Research Foundation.

Hoey, J., Montvernay, C. and Lambert, R. (1981) Wine and tobacco: risk factors for gastric cancer in France, *American Journal of Epidemiology* 113: 668–74.

Holst, P.A., Kromhout, D. and Brand, R. (1988) For debate: pet birds as an independent risk factor for lung cancer, *British Medical Journal* 297: 1319–21.

Hu, J.F., Zhang, S.F., Jia, E.M., Wang, Q.Q., Lin, S.D., Lin, Y.Y., Wu, Y.P. and Cheng, Y.T. (1988) Diet and cancer of the stomach: a case-control study in China, *International Journal of Cancer* 41: 331–5.

Infante, F., Voirol, M., Raymond, L., Hollenweger, V., Conti, M.C. and Loizeau, E. (1980) Alcohol, tobacco and nutriments consumption in liver cancer and cirrhosis patients in Geneva, *Les Colloques de l'INSERM* 95: 53–8.

International Agency for Research on Cancer (1988) *Alcohol drinking (monograph no. 44)*, Lyon: IARC.

Ishii, K., Takenchi, T. and Hirayama, T. (1973) Chronic calcifying pancreatitis and pancreatic carcinoma in Japan, *Digestion* 9: 429–37.

Jedrychowski, W., Wahrendorf, J., Popiela, T. and Rachtan, J. (1986) A case-control study of dietary factors and stomach cancer in Poland, *International Journal of Cancer* 37: 837–42.

Jensen, O.M. (1979) Cancer morbidity and causes of death among Danish brewery workers, *International Journal of Cancer* 23: 454–63.

Jensen, O.M. (1980) *Cancer morbidity and causes of death among Danish Brewery workers*, Lyon: IARC.

Kabat, G.C., Howson, C.P. and Wynder, E.L. (1986) Beer consumption and rectal cancer, *International Journal of Epidemiology* 15: 494–501.

Kaisary, A., Smith, P., Jaczq, E., McAllister, C.B., Wilkinson, G.R., Ray, W.A. and Branch, R.A. (1987) Genetic predisposition to bladder cancer: ability to hydroxylate debrisoquine and mephenytoin as risk factors, *Cancer Research* 47: 5488–93.

Katsouyanni, K., Trichopoulos, D., Boyle, P., Xirouchaki, E., Trichopoulou, A., Lisseos, B., Vasilaros, S. and McMahon, B. (1986) Diet and breast cancer: a case-control study in Greece, *International Journal of Cancer* 38: 815–20.

Keller, A.Z. and Terris, M. (1965) The association of alcohol and tobacco with cancer of the mouth and pharynx, *American Journal of Public Health* 55: 1578–85.

Klatsky, A.L., Friedman, G.D. and Siegelaub, A.B. (1981) Alcohol and mortality: a ten-year Kaiser-Permanente experience, *Annals of Internal Medicine* 95: 139–45.

Kodama, T. and Mori, W. (1983) Morphological lesions of the pancreatic ducts, *Acta Pathologica Japan* 33: 645–60.

Kono, S., Ikeda, M., Tokudome, S. and Nishizume, M. (1986) Alcohol and mortality: a cohort study of male Japanese physicians, *International Journal of Epidemiology* 15: 527–32.

Kune, S., Kune, G.A. and Watson, L.F. (1987) Case-control study of alcoholic beverages as etiological factors: the Melbourne colorectal cancer study, *Nutrition and Cancer* 9: 43–56.

Kvåle, G., Bjelke, E. and Gart, J.J. (1983) Dietary habits and lung cancer risk, *International Journal of Cancer* 31: 397–405.

Lam, K.C., Yu, M.C., Leung, J.W.C. and Henderson, B.E. (1982) Hepatitis B virus and cigarette-smoking: risk factors for hepatocellular carcinoma in Hong Kong, *Cancer Research* 42: 5246–8.

La Vecchia, C., Decarli, A., Franceschi, S., Pampallona, S. and Tognoni, G. (1985) Alcohol consumption and the risk of breast cancer in women, *Journal of the National Cancer Institute* 75: 61–5.

La Vecchia, C., Decarli, A., Franceschi, S., Gentile, A., Negri, E. and Parazzini, F. (1987) Dietary factors and the risk of breast cancer, *Nutrition and Cancer* 10: 205–14.

La Vecchia, C. and Negri, E. (1989) The role of alcohol in oesophageal cancer in non-smokers and of tobacco in non-drinkers, *International Journal of Cancer* 43: 784–5.

Le, M.G., Hill, C., Kramar, A. and Flamant, R. (1984) Alcohol beverage consumption and breast cancer in a French case-control study, *American Journal of Epidemiology* 120: 350–7.

Lin, R.S. and Kessler, I.I. (1981) A multifactorial model for pancreatic cancer in man: epidemiologic evidence, *Journal of the American Medical Association* 245: 147–52.

McDonald, W.C. and McDonald, J.B. (1987) Adenocarcinoma of the esophagus and/or gastric cardia, *Cancer* 60: 1094–8.

McMahon, B., Yen, S., Trichopoulos, D., Warren, K. and Nardi, G. (1981) Coffee and cancer of the pancreas, *New England Journal of Medicine* 304: 630–3.

Mack, T.M., Yu, M.C., Hanisch, R. and Henderson, B.E. (1986) Pancreas cancer and smoking, beverage consumption and past medical history, *Journal of the National. Cancer Institute* 76: 49–60.

Mandard, A.M., Duigon, F., Marnay, J., Masson, P., Qiu, S.L., Yu, J.S., Barrellier, P. and Lebigot, G. (1987) Analysis of the results of the micronucleus test in patients presenting upper digestive tract cancers and in non-cancerous subjects, *International Journal of Cancer* 39: 442–4.

Manousos, O., Papadimitriou, C., Trichopoulos, D., Polychronopoulou, A., Koutselinis, A. and Zavitsanos, X. (1981) Epidemiologic characteristics and trace elements in pancreatic cancer in Greece, *Cancer Detection and Prevention* 4: 439–42.

Martinez, I. (1969) Factors associated with cancers of the esophagus, mouth and pharynx in Puerto Rico, *Journal of the National Cancer Institute* 42: 1069–94.

Medina, E., Pascual, J.P., Medina, K.A.M. and Medina, R. (1983) Factors associated with occurrence of breast cancer in women in Chile: study of cases and controls, *Revista medica de Chile* 111: 1279–86.

Mettlin, C. (1989) Milk drinking, other beverage habits and lung cancer risk, *International Journal of Cancer* 43: 608–12.

Miller, A.B., Howe, G.R., Jain, M., Craib, K.J.P. and Harrison, L. (1983) Food items and food groups as risk factors in a case-control study of diet and colorectal cancer, *International Journal of Cancer* 32: 155–61.

Mommsen, S., Aagaard, J. and Sell, A. (1982) An epidemiological case-control study of bladder cancer in males from a predominantly rural district, *European Journal of Cancer and Clinical Oncology* 18: 1205–10.

Monson, R.R. and Lyon, J.L. (1975) Proportional mortality among alcoholics, *Cancer* 36: 1077–9.

Morgan, R.W. and Jain, M.G. (1974) Bladder cancer, smoking, beverages and artificial sweeteners, *Canadian Medical Association Journal* 111: 1067–70.

Nakachi, K., Imai, K., Hoshiyama, Y. and Sasaba, T. (1988) The joint effects of two factors in the aetiology of oesophageal cancer in Japan, *Journal of Epidemiology and Community Health* 42: 355–64.

Nielsen, M., Thomsen, J.L., Primdahl, S., Dyreborg, U. and Andersen, J.A. (1987) Breast cancer and atypia among young and middle-aged women: a study of 110 medicolegal autopsies, *British Journal of Cancer* 56: 814–19.

Norell, S.E., Ahlbom, A., Erwald, R., Jacobsen, G., Lindberg-Narior, I., Olin, R., Tornberg, B. and Wiechel, K.L. (1986) Diet and pancreatic cancer: a case-control study, *American Journal of Epidemiology* 124: 894–902.

Notani, P.N. (1988) Role of alcohol in cancers of the upper alimentary tract, use of models in risk assessment, *Journal of Epidemiology and Community Health* 42: 187–92.

O'Connell, D.L., Hulka, B.S., Chambless, L.E., Wilkinson, W.E. and Deubner, D.C. (1987) Cigarette-smoking, alcohol consumption and breast cancer risk, *Journal of the National Cancer Institute* 78: 229–34.

Office of Population Censuses and Surveys (1988) *Cancer statistics 1984: Registrations*, London: Her Majesty's Stationery Office.

Office of Population Censuses and Surveys (1989) *Mortality statistics: cause 1987*, London: Her Majesty's Stationery Office.

Olsen, J., Sabroe, S., Ipsen, J. (1985) Effect of combined alcohol and tobacco exposure on risk of cancer of the hypopharynx, *Journal of Epidemiology and Community Health* 39: 304–7.

Olsen, J., Sabroe, S. and Fasting, U. (1985) Interaction of alcohol and tobacco as risk factors in cancer of the laryngeal region, *Journal of Epidemiology and Community Health* 39: 165–8.

Oshima, A., Tsukuma, H., Hiyama, T., Fujimoto, I., Yamano, H. and Tanaka, M. (1984) Follow-up study of HBsAg-positive blood donors with special reference to effect of drinking and smoking on development of liver cancer, *International Journal of Cancer* 34: 775–9.

Paganini-Hill, A. and Ross, R.K. (1983) Breast cancer and alcohol consumption, *Lancet* ii: 626–7.

Pell, S. and D'Alonzo, C.A. (1973) A five-year mortality study of alcoholics, *Journal of Occupational Medicine* 15: 120–5.

Peto, R. (1985) The preventability of cancer, in Vessey, M.P. and Gray, M. (eds) *Cancer Risks and Prevention*, Oxford: Oxford University Press.

Pierce, R.J., Kune, G.A., Kune, S., Watson, L.F., Field, B., Merenstein, D., Hayes, A. and Irving, L.B. (1989) Dietary and alcohol intake, smoking pattern, occupational risk, and family history in lung cancer patients: results of a case control study in males, *Nutrition and Cancer* 12: 237–48.

Pollack, E.S., Nomura, A.M.Y., Heilbrun, L.K., Stemmerman, G.N. and Green, S.B. (1984) Prospective study of alcohol consumption and cancer, *New England Journal of Medicine* 310: 617–21.

Potter, J.D. and McMichael, A.J. (1986) Diet and cancer of the colon and rectum: a case-control study, *Journal of the National Cancer Institute* 76: 557–69.

Pottern, L.M., Morris, L.E., Blot, W.J., Ziegler, R.G. and Fraumeni, J.F. (1981) Esophageal cancer among black men in Washington DC, I: Alcohol, tobacco and other risk factors, *Journal of the National Cancer Institute* 67: 777–83.

Prior, P. (1988) Long-term cancer risk in alcoholism, *Alcohol and Alcoholism* 23: 163–71.

Risch, H.A., Burch, J.D., Miller, A.B., Hill, G.B., Steele. R. and Howe, G.R. (1988) Dietary factors and the incidence of cancer of the urinary bladder, *American Journal of Epidemiology* 127: 1179–91.

Robinette, C.D., Hrubec, Z. and Fraumeni, J.F. (1979) Chronic alcoholism and subsequent mortality in World War II veterans, *American Journal of Epidemiology* 109: 687–700.

Raymond, L., Infante, F., Tuyns, A.J., Voirol, M. and Lowenfelds, A.B. (1987) Diet and pancreatic cancer, *Gastroenterology and Clinical Biology* 11: 488–92.

Rohan, T.E. and McMichael, A.J. (1988) Alcohol consumption and the risk of breast cancer, *International Journal of Cancer* 41: 695–9.

Rosenberg, L., Stone, D., Shapiro, S., Kaufman, D.W., Helmrich, S.P., Miettinen, O.S., Stolley, P.D., Levy, M., Rosenshein, N.B., Schottenfeld, D. and Engle, R.L. (1982) Breast cancer and alcoholic beverage consuption, *Lancet* i: 267–71.

Sankaranarayanan, R., Duffy, S.W., Day, N.E., Krishnan Nair, M. and Padmakumary, G. (1989a) A case-control investigation of cancer of the oral tongue and the floor of the mouth in Southern India, *International Journal of Cancer* 44: 617–21.

Sankaranarayanan, R., Duffy, S.W., Padmakumary, G., Day, N.E. and Padmanabhan, T.K. (1989b) Tobacco chewing, alcohol and nasal snuff in cancer of the gingiva in Kerala, India, *British Journal of Cancer* 60: 638–43.

Schatzkin, A., Jones, D.Y., Hoover, R.N., Taylor, P.R., Brinton, L.A., Ziegler, R.G., Harvey, E.B., Carter, C.L., Licitra, L.M., Dufour, M.C. and Larson, D.B. (1987) Alcohol consumption and breast cancer in the epidemiologic follow-up study of the first National Health and Nutritional Examination Survey, *New England Journal of Medicine* 316: 1169–73.

Schatzkin, A., Piantadosi, S., Miccozzi, M. and Bartee, D. (1989a) Alcohol consumption and breast cancer: a cross-national correlation study, *International Journal of Epidemiology* 18: 28–31.

Schatzkin, A., Carter, C.L., Green, S.B., Kreger, B.E., Splansky, G.L., Anderson, K.M., Helsel, W.E. and Kannel, W.B. (1989b) Is alcohol consumption related to breast cancer? Results from the Framington Heart Study, *Journal of the National Cancer Institute* 81: 31–5.

Schmidt, W. and De Lint, J. (1972) Causes of death of alcoholics, *Quarterly Journal of Studies on Alcohol* 33: 171–85.

Schmidt, W. and Popham, R.E. (1981) The role of drinking and smoking in mortality from cancer and other causes in male alcoholics, *Cancer* 47: 1031–41.

Schwartz, D., Lellouch, J., Flamant, R. and Denoix, P.F. (1962) Alcohol and cancer: Results of a retrospective study, *Revue Francaise des Etudes Clinicales en Biologie* 7: 590–604.

Segal, I., Reinach, S.G. and de Beer, M. (1988) Factors associated with oesophageal cancer in Soweto, South Africa, *British Journal of Cancer* 58: 681–6.

Shibata, A., Hirohata, T., Toshima, H. and Tashiro, H. (1986) The role of drinking and cigarette smoking in the excess deaths from liver cancer, *Japanese Journal of Cancer Research (Gann)* 77: 287–95.

Slattery, M.L., Schumacher, M.C., West, D.W. and Robison, L.M. (1988) Smoking and bladder cancer: the modifying effect of cigarettes on other factors, *Cancer* 61: 402–8.

Smith, D.I. (1989) Relationship between alcohol consumption and breast cancer morbidity rates in Western Australia 1971–84, *Drug and Alcohol Dependence* 24: 61–5.

Smith, E.B. (1982) Epidemiology of cancers of the oral cavity and pharynx. in Correa, P. and Haenszel, W. (eds) *Epidemiology of cancer of the digestive tract*, The Hague: Martinus Nijhoff.

Spalajkovic, M. (1976) Alcoholism and cancer of the larynx and hypopharynx, *Journal Francais de l'Oto-rhino-laryngologie* 25: 49–50.

Stemhagen, A., Slade, J., Altman, R. and Bill, J. (1983) Occupational risk factors and liver cancer: a retrospective case-control study of primary liver cancer in New Jersey, *American Journal of Epidemiology* 117: 443–54.

Stocks, P. (1957) Cancer incidence in North Wales and Liverpool region in relation to habits and environment, in *British Empire Cancer Campaign 35th Annual Report, Part II (suppl.)*, London.

Sundby, P. (1967) *Alcoholism and mortality*, Oslo: Universitetsforlaget.

Talamini, R., La Vecchia, C., Decarli, A., Franceschi, S., Grattoni, E., Grigletto, E., Liberati, A. and Tognoni, G. (1984) Social factors, diet and breast cancer in a Northern Italian population, *British Journal of Cancer* 49: 723–9.

Thomas, D.B., Uhl, C.N. and Hartge, P. (1983) Bladder cancer and alcoholic beverage consumption, *American Journal of Epidemiology* 118: 720–7.

Tricholopoulos, D., Ouranos, G., Day, N.E., Tzonou, A., Manousos, O., Papadimitriou, C. and Tricholopoulos, A. (1985) Diet and cancer of the stomach: a case-control study in Greece, *International Journal of Cancer* 36: 291–7.

Trichopoulos, D., Day, N.E., Kaklamani, E., Tzonou, A., Munoz, N., Zavitsanos, X., Koumantaki, Y. and Trichopoulos, A. (1987) Hepatitis B virus, tobacco-smoking and ethanol consumption in the etiology of hepatocellular carcinomas, *International Journal of Cancer* 39: 45–9.

Tuyns, A.J., Esteve, J., Raymond, L., Berrino, F., Benhamon, E., Blanchet, F., Boffeta, P., Cronignomi, P., Del Moral, A., Lehmann, W., Merletti, F., Pequignot, G., Riboli, E., Sancho-Garnier, H., Terracinic, B., Zubiri, A. and Zubiri, Z. (1988) Cancer of the larynx/hypopharynx, tobacco and alcohol, *International Journal of Cancer* 41: 483–91.

Tuyns, A.J., Pequignot, G. and Jensen, O.M. (1977) Oesophageal cancer in Ille-et-Vilaine in relation to alcohol and tobacco consumption: multiplicative risks, *Bulletin of Cancer* 64: 45–60.

Tuyns, A.J., Pequignot, G. and Abbatucci, J.S. (1979) Oesophageal cancer and alcohol consumption: importance of type of beverage, *International Journal of Cancer* 23: 443–7.

Tuyns, A.J., Pequignot, G., Gignoux, M. and Valla, A. (1982) Cancers of the digestive tract, alcohol and tobacco, *International Journal of Cancer* 30: 9–11.

Ubukata, T., Oshima, A., Morinaga, K., Hirayama, T., Kamiyama, S., Shimada, A. and Kim, J.P. (1987) Cancer patterns among Koreans in Japan, Koreans in Korea and Japanese in Japan in relation to lifestyle factors, *Japanese Journal of Cancer Research* 78: 437–46.

Vassallo, A., Correa, P., De Stefani, E., Cendan, M., Zarala, D., Chen, V., Carsioglo, J. and Dereo-Pellegrini, H. (1985) Oesophageal cancer in Uruguay: a case-control study, *Journal of the National Cancer Institute* 75: 1005–9.

Victoria, C.G., Munoz, N., Day, N.E., Barcelos, L.B., Peccin, D.A. and Braga, N.M. (1987) Hot beverages and oesophageal cancer in Southern Brazil: a case-control study, *International Journal of Cancer* 39: 710–16.

Vincent, R.G. and Marchetta, F. (1963) The relationship of the use of tobacco and alcohol to cancer of the oral cavity, pharynx or larynx, *American Journal of Surgery* 106: 501–5.

Webster, L.A., Layde, P.M., Wingo, P.A. and Dry, H.W. (1983) Alcohol consumption and risk of breast cancer, *Lancet* ii: 724–6.

Willett, W.C., Stampfer, M.J., Colditz, G.A., Rosner, B.A., Hennekens, C.H. and Speizer, F.E. (1987) Moderate alcohol consumption and the risk of breast cancer, *New England Journal of Medicine* 316: 1174–80.

Williams, R.R. and Horm, J.W. (1977) Association of cancer sites with tobacco and alcohol consumption and socioeconomic status of patients: interview study from the Third National Cancer Survey, *Journal of the National Cancer Institute* 58: 525–47.

Woolf, B. (1955) On estimating the relationship between blood group and disease, *Annals of Human Genetics* 19: 251–3.

Wu, A.H., Paganini-Hill, A., Ross, R.K. and Henderson, B.E. (1987) Alcohol, physical activity and other risk factors for colorectal cancer: a prospective study, *British Journal of Cancer* 55: 687–94.

Wynder, E.L. and Bross, I.J. (1961) A study of etiological factors in cancer of the oeso-phagus, *Cancer* 14: 389–413.

Wynder, E.L., Bross, I.J. and Day, E. (1956) A study of environmental factors in cancer of the larynx, *Cancer* 9: 86–110.

Wynder, E.L., Bross, I.J. and Feldman, R.M. (1957) A study of etiological factors in cancer of the mouth, *Cancer* 10: 1300–23.

Wynder, E.L., Corey, L.S., Mabuchi, K. and Mushinski, M. (1976) Environmental factors in cancer of the larynx: a second look, *Cancer* 38: 1591–601.

Wynder, E.L., Kmet, J., Dungal, N. and Segi, M. (1963) An epidemiological investigation of gastric cancer, *Cancer* 16: 1461–97.

Wynder, E.L. and Shigematsu, T. (1967) Environmental factors of cancer of the colon and rectum, *Cancer* 20: 1520–61.

Wynder, E.L., Mabuchi, K., Maruchi, N. and Fortner, J.G. (1973) A case-control study of cancer of the pancreas, *Cancer* 31: 641–8.

Wynder, E.L., Hall, N.E.L. and Polansky, M. (1983) Epidemiology of coffee and pan-creatic cancer, *Cancer Research* 43: 3900–6.

Wynder, E.L., Onderdonk, J. and Mantel, N. (1963) An epidemiological investigation of cancer of the bladder, *Cancer* 16: 1388–407.

Young, T.B. (1989) A case-control study of breast cancer and alcohol consumption habits, *Cancer* 64: 552–8.

Yu, M.C., Mack, T., Hanisch, R., Peters, R.L., Henderson, B.E. and Pike, M.C. (1983) Hepatitis, alcohol consumption, cigarette-smoking and hepatocellular carcinoma in Los Angeles, *Cancer Research* 43: 6077–9.

Yu, M.C., Garabrant, D.H., Peters, J.M. and Mack, T.M. (1988) Tobacco, alcohol, diet, occupation and carcinoma of the esophagus, *Cancer Research* 48: 3843–8.

Zagraniski, R.T., Kelsey, J.L. and Walter, S.D. (1986) Occupational risk factors for laryngeal carcinoma, Connecticut, 1975–80, *American Journal of Epidemiology* 124: 67–76.

7 Alcohol and Damage to the Foetus and Reproductive System

This chapter provides a brief review of research in the area of alcohol consumption and its effect on the reproductive system in both sexes and on the foetus. In contrast to the effects on the reproductive system, there is considerable research about the impact on the foetus, including case reports and prospective cohort epidemiological surveys attempting to distinguish the causal contribution of alcohol to various birth defects. There has been little emphasis on developing indicators of either incidence or prevalence of these types of harm.

7.1 Clinical problems

7.1.1 Effects on the male reproductive system

Reported effects of chronic alcohol abuse on the reproductive system include loss of libido, damaged testicular function, infertility, impotence, hypogonadism (secretory deficiency of the gonads) and gynaecomastia (abnormal enlargement of the male breast). Although these are often sequelae of liver cirrhosis, they have been reported among alcoholics without liver disease (van Thiel and Lester, 1974). It is believed that liver dysfunction is partly responsible for these effects, but also that ethanol per se is a gonadal toxin and a direct cause of testicular damage (Lindholm et al., 1978).

Up to 50% of chronic heavy drinkers complain of loss of libido (Morgan and Pratt, 1982). The other problems appear to be considerably rarer. Lemere and Smith (1973) reported impotence in 8% of chronic alcoholics in a series of about 17,000 cases. Of these, about 50% remained impotent even after long periods of abstinence from alcohol.

Again regarding testicular function, Lindholm et al. (1978), reporting on a series of 30 alcoholics, noted normal spermatogenesis in 12 men, severely reduced spermatogenesis in 9 and gynaecomastia in 1, and remarked that 50% of the men had smaller testes than normal. The meaning of this latter finding is obscure, since one would normally not be surprised with any group to find that 50% of them were below average on whatever characteristic was being examined. These men were all long-established heavy drinkers, with drinking careers of 10–40 years in duration involving the daily consumption of between 150 and 200 grams of ethanol – about 18–24 standard drinks per day. It is difficult to generalise from such a small sample, or to assess the causal influence of ethanol consumption in association with other factors on the observed disorders.

Although Morgan and Pratt (1982) reported that of 90 men attending an infertility clinic 40% were 'thought' (sic) to have reduced sperm counts as a result of drinking 4–6 units of alcohol per day, larger controlled studies lend little credence to this speculation.

Buiatti et al. (1984), reporting on a case-control study of 112 azoospermic or oligospermic males and 127 controls in Italy, found no association with alcohol consumption. Marshburn et al. (1989) studied 546 men in an infertility clinic, although the effective sample size was reduced to 445 following exclusion of men with physical injury and disease. They found no association between alcohol consumption and volume of sperm, sperm density, motility, motile density and the proportions of dead or damaged sperm.

In short, the association between chronic heavy drinking and damage to the reproductive system in men is clearly established. Overall, there is no reason to believe that moderate levels of drinking incur significant risks to the reproductive system or to fertility.

7.1.2 Effects on the female reproductive system

Less research has been performed in this area, probably because of the relatively small numbers of female chronic alcoholics, and also the comparative difficulty of clinical investigation. Amenorrhoea, anovulation, luteal phase dysfunction and ovarian pathology have been noted in alcohol-dependent women, but there are no reliable estimates of the prevalence of these disorders (Mello et al., 1989).

In non-alcohol-dependent women, associations between alcohol consumption and menstrual disorders have ben reported. Mendelson et al. (1988) reported an experiment in which 26 women volunteers were observed in a clinical ward setting for several weeks. This sample size is too small to produce statistically detectable associations, and the study also failed to make any attempt to control for confounding factors or baseline characteristics of the women. Wilsnack et al. (1984) reported associations between drinking and dysmenorrhoea, heavy menstrual flow and premenstrual discomfort in a US survey of 917 women. These were particularly strongly associated with drinking 6 or more drinks (US) per day at least once a week. However, other risk factors were not controlled for.

Olsen et al. (1983) studied 1,069 infertile couples from an infertility clinic in Denmark, and compared them with a control group of 4,305 fertile couples. They concluded that moderate alcohol consumption did not appear to play a role in the development of subfecundity. Wilcox et al. (1988) also failed to find an association between alcohol consumption and the probability of becoming pregnant in a given menstrual cycle among a sample of 104 women who had been attempting to become pregnant for 3 months.

To sum up then, chronic heavy drinking in women leads to reproductive system damage and menstrual dysfunction. It seems possible that menstrual dysfunction may also occur at lower levels of consumption, but there are no studies establishing a causal relationship at low levels or attempting estimation of the levels of risk involved.

7.2 Effects on the foetus

Alcohol is associated with a continuum of birth damage, which may be very serious or relatively inconsequential (Barrison et al., 1985). At the most serious extreme is a combination of developmental delay, growth retardation, neurological abnormalities and characteristic facial dysmorphology known as the Foetal Alcohol Syndrome (FAS). Other damage, including physical abnormalities, developmental delays and foetal growth retardation are known as Foetal Alcohol Effects (FAE).

Heavy alcohol consumption during pregnancy (over 56 units a week) can result in a child being born with FAS (Barrison et al., 1985). Follow-up studies in the United States have demonstrated that the effects are permanent (Streissguth et al., 1985). However, both American and British experiences show that only about 2.5% of very heavy-drinking mothers produce such infants (Abel, 1984). But although not all the offspring of very heavy drinking mothers exhibit the full-blown FAS, many show signs of damage, for example craniofacial abnormalities (Rostand et al., 1990). Abel (1984) has estimated that about 10% show some signs of damage. Indeed, in one Belfast survey of such offspring, only 1 out of 23 was normal (Halliday, 1982).

The exact teratogenic mechanism of FAS remains unclear but is obviously not solely dependent on alcohol (Foster, 1986). Experimental studies in animals point to mineral deficiency, particularly zinc, which in combination with alcohol intake may lead to serious birth defects (Porter et al., 1984). However, some women who have produced children with the syndrome have normal plasma zinc levels (Halmesmaki, 1985). American experience suggests that FAS is more commonly found among the offspring of very heavy-drinking mothers who are also socially and materially deprived (Bingol et al., 1988). Confusion over the relative contribution of alcohol in causing this syndrome has led to the suggestion that titles such as 'Foetal Poverty Syndrome' or 'Foetal Alcohol Lifestyle Syndrome' may be more appropriate than Foetal Alcohol Syndrome (Zuckerman et al., 1986). However, although the relative contribution of alcohol may eventually be shown to be less than that of other variables, the fact that reduction of intake in alcoholic women has been of demonstrable benefit to their offspring (Little et al., 1978) suggests that heavy drinking remains an integral factor.

More moderate but regular levels of intake have been associated with a wide variety of foetal problems, such as an increased incidence of stillbirths, spontaneous abortions, pre-term delivery, morphological abnormalities, growth retardation and delayed mental development (Barrison et al., 1985; Plant, 1985). Some of these findings are also controversial. Many studies have failed to take account of the timing, amount and type of alcohol, or to distinguish the effects of regular from binge drinking (Day, 1991; Knupfer, 1991). Others have not distinguished the specific effects of alcohol from other confounding influences known to affect pregnancy outcome, such as social class, smoking, diet, ethnic status, parity, drug use or maternal age (Zuckerman and Hingson, 1986). Smoking may exacerbate the effects of alcohol (Wright et al., 1983; Plant, 1985; Plant, 1988; Brooke et al., 1989).

The most robust finding is an association of alcohol consumption in excess of the comparatively low level of 10 units per week, in the early stages of pregnancy with a significant risk of reduced birth weight. This has been demonstrated in studies carried out in London (Wright et al., 1983; Little et al., 1986; Brooke et al., 1989) and in Scotland (Plant, 1985; Sulaiman et al., 1988). Only one British study has commented on relative risks. Wright et al. (1983) found a statistically significant relative risk of birth-weight less than the 10th centile of 2.27 in women consuming more than 10 units of alcohol per week in the early stages of pregnancy as compared with those drinking less than 5 units. Further evidence for this conclusion comes from studies illustrating that a reduction of intake in pregnancy, particularly if started in the first trimester, is associated with improved foetal growth (Halmesmaki, 1988).

Low birthweight remains the most potent predictor of childhood mortality, morbidity and impaired later development (National Children's Bureau, 1987) but there is no general agreement about the relative importance of contributory factors. It is clear that the impact of alcohol on birthweight is less than that of other factors. Sulaiman et al. (1988) found that alcohol consumption accounted for no more than 2.5% of the variation in birth weight and Plant (1985) 0.5%.

Adverse developmental outcomes appear to be related to higher consumption throughout pregnancy. Long-term follow-up studies have detected an effect on growth and mental performance at 3 years (Day et al., 1991) and at 7 years (Streissguth et al., 1990) when mothers were drinking more than 30 units of alcohol per week.

In conclusion, drinking more than 56 units of alcohol a week may result in a child with FAS or with some damage (FAE). Drinking in excess of 30 units a week is linked with developmental problems and drinking in excess of 10 units a week with a reduction in birthweight. Some researchers have suggested that there is no evidence that these effects are seen at very low levels of intake (Roman, 1988; Knupfer, 1991). Others have said that there is no conclusive proof that low levels of drinking are harmless, arguing that since there is an enormous range of harms related to pre-natal alcohol exposure, it seems unlikely that there is any single definite threshold of harmless alcohol intake.

7.3 The extent of these problems in the United Kingdom

Any useful consideration of absolute risk is dependent on reliable data about the prevalence and incidence of cases. It also requires data about the prevalence of alcoholism, chronic heavy drinking and drinking levels among men, non-pregnant and pregnant women. Suitable data are rare and incomplete.

7.3.1 Damage to the reproductive system

Chronic alcoholics and heavy drinkers form a small proportion of the population and are difficult to identify. So it is perhaps not surprising that it is not possible to locate any epidemiological or population studies which attempt to estimate the prevalence of alcohol-related damage to the reproductive system in either men or women.

7.3.2 Damage to the foetus

Although the criteria for FAS are clear (Barrison et al., 1985), diagnosis can be problematic. There are no biochemical or other tests such as are available for other handicapping conditions, e.g. Down's Syndrome. Diagnosis is dependent on retrospective questioning about maternal drinking during pregnancy, and there may be difficulties in obtaining accurate information. Furthermore, even when diagnosis is clear, FAS is not a notifiable condition and therefore does not appear as a separate classification in any routine records of infant morbidity. Despite British case reports of FAS (Poskitt et al., 1982; Beattie et al., 1983), it appears to be rare in the United Kingdom In contrast to experience abroad, no British prospective sample of pregnant women has so far identified any (Wright et al., 1983; Plant, 1985; Little, 1986; Sulaiman et al., 1988; Brooke et al., 1989).

Less than 1% of women of child-bearing age consume in excess of 56 units of alcohol per week (Breeze, 1985; Goddard and Ikin, 1988). We do not know how many of them become pregnant. The only idea of incidence of FAS that is available is based on extrapolation from epidemiological studies of pregnant women. One such report based on 20 studies from Australia, North America and Europe suggests a worldwide incidence for FAS of 1.9 per 1,000 live births, compared with an incidence of roughly 1.25 for Down's Syndrome and 1.0 for spina bifida (Abel and Sokol, 1987). Live births in the United Kingdom in 1988 totalled 787,600 (Central Statistical Office, 1989). Applying this ratio of 1.9 cases per 1,000 births would yield an incidence of 1,496 cases of FAS in the United Kingdom in 1988. This is a far higher incidence than the frequency of published clinical case reports would suggest.

Assessing the impact of FAE is even more difficult. In diagnosis, the effects of alcohol such as low birthweight are indistinguishable from the effects of other confounding influences. Consequently, there are no specific data on case prevalence.

In England and Wales, about 1% of women of all ages drink more than 30 units of alcohol a week, and 15% of women (Breeze, 1985) and 22% of women under 44 years (Goddard and Ikin, 1988) drink more than 10 units of alcohol a week. These data pertain to all women, not just those who are pregnant. Surveys of drinking levels among pregnant women offer inconsistent data. In a West London survey, 19% were consuming more than 10 units of alcohol a week (Waterson and Murray-Lyon, 1989), but 13% were reported in a Midlands study (Davis et al., 1982), and 5.7% in a Scottish study (Plant, 1985). Any calculation of absolute risk among these women would also need to take account of the prevalence of other confounding variables, and such data are unavailable.

7.4 Conclusion

Very heavy alcohol use is associated with damage to the reproductive system in both males and females and with foetal damage. More moderate drinking is associated with foetal damage and probably with menstrual disorders in women. It is impossible to gauge with any accuracy the prevalence or incidence of such damage in the United Kingdom.

References

Abel, E.L. (1984) *Fetal Alcohol Syndrome and Fetal Alcohol Effects*, Vol. 1, New York: Plenum Press.

Abel, E.L. and Sokol, R. (1987) Incidence of Fetal Alcohol Syndrome and economic impact of FAS-related anomalies, *Drug and Alcohol Dependence* 19: 51–70.

Barrison, I.G., Waterson, E.J. and Murray-Lyon, I.M. (1985) Adverse effects of alcohol in pregnancy, *British Journal of Addiction* 80: 11–22.

Beattie, J.O., Day, R.E., Cockburn, F. and McClure, G. (1983) Alcohol and the fetus in the west of Scotland, *British Medical Journal* 287: 17–19.

Bingol, N., Schuster, C., Fuchs, M., Aosub, S., Turner, G., Stone, R.K. and Gromisch, D.S. (1987) The influence of socioeconomic factors on the occurrence of Fetal Alcohol Syndrome, *Advances in Alcohol and Substance Abuse* 6: 105–18.

Breeze, E. (1985) *Women and Drinking*, London: HMSO.

Brooke, O.G., Anderson, H.R., Bland, J.M., Peacock, B.L. and Stewart, C.M. (1989) Effects on birthweight of smoking, alcohol, caffeine, socio-economic factors and psychosocial stress, *British Medical Journal* 298: 795–801.

Buiatti, E., Barchielli, A., Geddes, M., Nastasi, L., Kriebel, D., Franchini, M. and Scarselli, G. (1984) Risk factors in male infertility: a case-control study, *Archives of Environmental Health* 39: 266–70.

Central Statistical Office (1989) *Monthly Digest of Statistics* No. 528, London: HMSO.

Davis, P.J., Partridge, J.W. and Storrs, C.N. (1982) Alcohol consumption in pregnancy. How much is safe?, *Archives of Disease in Childhood* 57: 940–3.

Day, N.L. (1991) Methodological problems in measuring harm, *British Journal of Addiction* 86: 1057–9.

Day, N.L., Robles, N., Richardson, G., Geva, D., Taylor, P., Scher, M., Stoffer, D., Cornelius, M. and Goldschmidt, L. (1991) The effects of prenatal alcohol use on the growth of children at three years of age, *Alcoholism: Clinical and Experimental Research* 15: 67–71.

Foster, J.W. (1986) Possible maternal auto-immune component in the etiology of Fetal Alcohol Syndrome, *Developmental Medicine and Child Neurology* 28: 649–61.

Goddard, E. and Ikin, C. (1988) *Drinking in England and Wales 1987*, London: HMSO.

Halliday, H.L., Reid, M. and McClure, G. (1982) Results of heavy drinking in pregnancy, *British Journal of Obstetrics and Gynaecology* 84: 892–5.

Halmesmaki, E., Ylikorkala, O. and Alftan, G. (1985) Concentrations of zinc and copper in pregnant problem drinkers and their newborn infants, *British Medical Journal* 291: 1470–1.

Halmesmaki, E. (1988) Alcohol counselling of 85 pregnant problem drinkers: effect on drinking and fetal outcome, *British Journal of Obstetrics and Gynaecology* 95: 243–7.

Jones, K.L., Smith, D.W., Streissguth, A.P. and Myrianthopoulos, N.C. (1974) Outcome in offspring of chronic alcoholic women, *Lancet* i: 1076–8.

Knupfer, G. (1991) Abstaining for fetal health: the fiction that even light drinking is dangerous, *British Journal of Addiction* 86: 1063–74.

Lemere, F. and Smith, J.W. (1973) Alcohol-induced sexual impotence, *American Journal of Psychiatry* 130: 212–13.

Lindholm, J., Fabricius-Bjerre, N., Bahnsen, M., Boiesen, P., Bangstrup, L., Pedersen, M.L. and Hagen, C. (1978) Pituitary testicular function in patients with chronic alcoholism, *European Journal of Clinical Investigation* 8: 269–72.

Little, R.E. and Streissguth, A.P. (1978) Drinking during pregnancy in alcoholic women, *Alcoholism* 2: 179–82.

Little, R.E., Asker, R.L., Sampson, P. and Renwick, B.H. (1986) Fetal growth and moderate drinking in early pregnancy, *American Journal of Epidemiology* 123: 270–8.

Marshburn, P.B., Sloan, C.S. and Hammond, M.G. (1989) Semen quality and association with coffee-drinking, cigarette-smoking and alcohol consumption, *Fertility and Sterility* 52: 161–5.

Mello, N.K., Mendelson, J.H. and Teoh, S.K. (1989) Neuroendocrine consequences of alcohol abuse in women, *Annals of the New York Academy of Science* 562: 211–40.

Mendelson, J.H. and Mello, N. (1988) Chronic alcohol effects on anterior pituitary and ovarian hormones in healthy women, *Journal of Pharmacology and Experimental Therapeutics* 245: 407–12.

Morgan, M. and Pratt, O.E. (1982) Sex, alcohol and the developing fetus, *British Medical Bulletin* 38: 43–52.

National Children's Bureau (1987) *Child Health Ten Years After the Court Report: Where are the Child Health Services Going?*, London: National Children's Bureau.

Olsen, J., Rachootin, P., Schidt, A.V. and Damsbo, N. (1983) Tobacco use, alcohol consumption and infertility, *International Journal of Epidemiology* 12: 179–84.

Plant, M. (1985) *Women, Drinking and Pregnancy* London: Tavistock.

Plant, M.D. and Plant, M.A. (1988) Maternal use of alcohol and other drugs during pregnancy and birth abnormalities: further results from a prospective study, *Alcohol and Alcoholism* 23: 229–233.

Poikolainen, K. (1991) Abstain from poisoning your unborn child, *British Journal of Addiction* 86: 1060–1.

Porter, R., O'Connor, M. and Whelan, J. (eds) (1984) *Mechanisms of Alcohol Damage in Utero* (Ciba Symposium No. 105), London: Pitman.

Poskitt, E.M.E., Hersey, O.J. and Smith, C.S. (1982) Alcohol, other drugs and the fetus, *Developmental Medicine and Child Neurology* 24: 596–602.

Roman, P.M. (1988) Biological features of women's alcohol use: a review, *Public Health* 103: 628–37.

Rostand, A., Kaminski, M., Lelong, N., Dehane, P., Delestre, I., Lein-Bernard, C., Querleu, D. and Crepin, G. (1990) Alcohol use in pregnancy, craniofacial features, and fetal growth, *Journal of Epidemiology and Community Health* 44: 302–6.

Streissguth, A.P., Clarren, S.K. and Jones, K.L. (1985) Natural history of the Foetal Alcohol Syndrome: a ten-year follow-up of eleven patients, *Lancet* ii: 85–91.

Streissguth, A.P., Barr, H.M. and Sampson, P.D. (1990) Moderate prenatal alcohol exposure: effects on child IQ and learning problems at age seven and a half years, *Alcoholism: Clinical and Experimental Research* 14: 662–9.

Sulaiman, N., Florey, C. du V. and Taylor, D. (1988) Alcohol consumption in Dundee primigravidas and its effects on outcome of pregnancy, *British Medical Journal* 296: 1500–3.

van Thiel, D.H. and Lester, R. (1974) Sex and alcohol, *New England Journal of Medicine* 291: 251–3.

Waterson, E.J. and Murray-Lyon, I.M. (1989) Drinking and smoking patterns amongst women attending an antenatal clinic – I: before pregnancy, *Alcohol and Alcoholism* 24: 153–62.

Wilcox, A., Weinberg, C. and Baird, D. (1988) Caffeinated beverages and decreased fertility, *Lancet* ii: 1453–6.

Wilsnack, S.C., Klassen, A.D. and Wilsnack, R.W. (1984) Drinking and reproductive dysfunction among women in a 1981 national survey, *Alcohol and Alcoholism* 8: 451–8.

Wright, J.T., Waterson, E.J., Barrison, I.G., Toplis, P., Lewis, I.G., Gordon, M., MacRae, K.D., Morris, N.F. and Murray-Lyon, I.M. (1983) Alcohol consumption, pregnancy and low birthweight, *Lancet* i: 663–5.

Zuckerman, B.S. and Hingson, R. (1986) Alcohol consumption during pregnancy: a critical review, *Developmental Medicine and Child Neurology* 28: 649–61.

8 Alcohol and Non-malignant Gastrointestinal Disease

The major contributor to morbidity and mortality from this group of diseases is pancreatitis. Research reports in this field are difficult to interpret because the diagnostic criteria for pancreatitis are not used consistently across studies. Estimates of the incidence of acute pancreatitis vary widely across studies, but rates of around 100 cases per million population per year may be reasonable. Mortality rates increase with age, rising from around 20 per million per year at age 40–45 to over 40 per million per year at age 60–65 for men; the equivalent figures for women are 5 and 20. By age 80–85, women's mortality exceeds men's, with both being over 100 per million per year. Although there is very clear evidence of the importance of alcohol consumption as a causative factor for some forms of pancreatitis, it is not clear from the published research how much of either the morbidity or mortality due to pancreatitis can be attributed to alcohol. Comparing diseases of the pancreas with those of the liver, it seems that diseases of the pancreas attributable to alcohol may contribute more to acute hospital admissions, but alcoholic liver disease is a much commoner cause of death. Alcohol is also implicated in chronic gastritis. However, there seems to be no published work which quantifies this.

8.1 Non-malignant gastrointestinal disease

The conditions considered under this heading are:

1. Oesophageal disorders
2. Peptic ulcers – gastric and duodenal
3. Gastritis
4. Coeliac disease
5. Crohn's disease
6. Ulcerative colitis
7. Pancreatic disease

For conditions 1, 4, 5 and 6, there is no evidence or reason to consider alcohol as a risk factor. The position is less clear for ulcers and gastritis. There is evidence that alcohol consumption is greater in patients with peptic ulcers. However, it is associated with other risk factors for ulcer, such as smoking and emotional stress, and does not emerge as an independent risk factor in multivariate analysis (Walker et al. (1988) is a recent study in

Table 8.1: Mortality from diseases of the pancreas, 1979–88

Scotland

Age group	25–	30–	35–	40–	45–	50–	55–	60–	65–	70–	75–	80–	85+
MEN													
Total deaths	7	10	19	31	29	36	47	41	42	57	60	29	21
Rate/million/yr	4	6	11	21	21	26	34	34	41	68	110	111	184
WOMEN													
Total deaths	3	7	4	8	16	15	21	31	44	70	79	79	63
Rate/million/yr	2	4	2	5	11	10	14	22	33	58	81	128	159

England and Wales

Age group	25–	30–	35–	40–	45–	50–	55–	60–	65–	70–	75–	80–	85+
MEN													
Total deaths	32	86	117	164	173	240	337	450	508	587	557	392	252
Rate/million/yr	2	5	7	11	12	18	24	35	47	66	94	132	180
WOMEN													
Total deaths	14	34	59	73	85	123	169	313	498	624	775	827	850
Rate/million/yr	1	2	3	5	6	9	12	22	38	52	79	128	188

this area). Some studies have found that continued alcohol use inhibits the healing of peptic ulcers (e.g. Reynolds et al., 1989), whereas other large prospective studies (e.g. Naisry et al., 1987) have found no such association. Again, the positive results could be the result of confounding from other inhibitors of healing. Overall, the medical consensus is that alcohol plays no part in the aetiology of gastric or duodenal ulcers.

The term 'gastritis' is used to describe disorders of the lining of the gastrointestinal tract. It is usually diagnosed by endoscopy for gastrointestinal bleeding. The literature contains several case studies, which indicate that certain types of gastritis (particularly 'atrophic gastritis' and 'haemorrhagic gastritis') are predominantly diseases of chronic alcohol abuse (e.g. Segawa et al., 1988; Laine, 1988). However, there do not seem to be any reports which would make it possible to quantify the extent of this problem.

Alcohol is well established as an important risk factor for pancreatic disease. The disease is frequently classified into 'alcoholic', 'biliary' and 'idiopathic'. As we will see below, this classification is not helpful in establishing the role of alcohol in its aetiology. The remainder of this chapter will review the evidence on the morbidity and mortality from pancreatic disease in relation to alcohol consumption.

8.2 Mortality from pancreatic disease

Table 8.1 gives the mortality from pancreatic diseases (underlying cause of death no. 577) from the Annual Reports of the Registrar General for

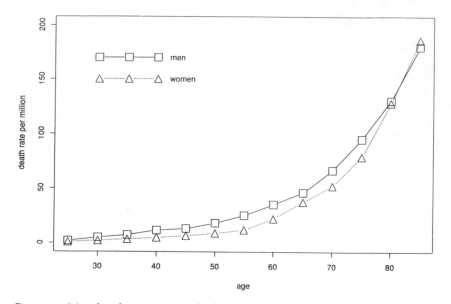

Figure 8.1 Mortality from pancreatic diseases. (Source: Annual Reports of the Registrar
General for Scotland and the Office of Population Censuses and Surveys for England and
Wales 1979–88.)

Scotland and the Office of Population Censuses and Surveys for England
and Wales over the period 1979–88, and the combined data are plotted in
Figure 8.1.

These deaths are subdivided into two categories: 577.0, acute pancreatitis, and 577.1, chronic pancreatitis. They are not separately listed in the
Scottish data, but the English figures show that acute pancreatitis accounts
for fewer than 10% of deaths in men and fewer than 7% of the deaths in
women. The proportion of deaths due to acute pancreatitis is higher at
younger ages. More than 20% of deaths due to pancreatic disease for men
under 50 are classified as acute pancreatitis.

Death rates for men exceed those for women at the younger age groups.
The English and Scottish rates are similar except for males aged 35–60,
where the English rates are lower than those for Scotland.

During this ten-year period, the same coding system (ninth revision of
the International Classification of Diseases) was used for causes of death.
The only substantial change recorded with the use of these codes occurred
in 1984 when a new WHO 3 rule was implemented in the coding of deaths.
This instructed the coders to look for an underlying cause of death among
subsequent information on a death certificate, for certain causes of death
such as bronchopneumonia, which could take precedence over that assigned
by the doctor completing the form. A double coding exercise undertaken
in 1984 suggested that this might result in an 8% increase in rate for cause

Table 8.2: Death rates per million (cause 577) by age group and year, England and Wales

MALES

						Age group							
	25–	30–	35–	40–	45–	50–	55–	60–	65–	70–	75–	80–	85+
1979	2	7	8	10	14	21	26	41	45	66	81	122	160
1980	1	3	12	7	17	19	37	43	46	51	104	128	131
1981	4	7	9	8	12	23	21	45	36	65	115	119	135
1982	2	6	8	11	9	20	27	37	45	77	64	164	171
1983	1	5	4	12	14	13	18	35	48	58	93	128	128
1984	1	4	7	10	14	10	20	35	49	74	100	132	226
1985	1	5	5	18	10	23	25	35	47	59	95	174	231
1986	2	5	8	12	8	16	23	25	58	57	85	120	201
1987	3	5	5	6	15	11	20	28	46	86	109	99	151
1988	1	3	4	13	12	19	26	32	48	72	93	136	236

FEMALES

						Age group							
	25–	30–	35–	40–	45–	50–	55–	60–	65–	70–	75–	80–	85+
1979	4	1	3	7	7	12	19	33	37	42	69	121	155
1980	1	2	3	4	4	11	11	26	36	42	80	125	112
1981	0	1	1	6	7	10	12	23	36	49	67	124	200
1982	1	2	8	5	6	12	10	20	40	56	77	95	171
1983	0	1	3	7	5	12	10	20	41	48	60	119	195
1984	1	2	4	3	7	7	10	18	50	55	94	118	145
1985	0	3	2	3	6	4	15	19	37	52	103	123	223
1986	1	2	4	5	7	6	9	20	47	66	79	144	219
1987	1	4	2	5	6	9	9	21	28	48	83	151	213
1988	1	2	5	4	7	5	12	24	30	58	75	152	220

of death 577. Age-specific death rates for England and Wales by year of death are given in Table 8.2.

In the oldest age-groups (80 years and older), the mortality rates appear to increase somewhat from 1984 onwards (possibly as a result of WHO 3). In the younger age groups, there are few apparent trends over this ten-year period. There is a suggestion of a decrease in death rates for the 60–65 age group for both sexes, but it is not very marked.

8.3 Acute or chronic pancreatic disease

Pancreatitis is usually classified as either chronic or acute. This is not really a diagnostic criterion, but only a classification of the way in which the disease presents (Sarles et al., 1989). Another interpretation is to suggest that acute pancreatitis is a manifestation of chronic pancreatitis. In acute pancreatitis, patients generally present with acute abdominal pain. The diagnosis is then confirmed by examining the pathology of the pancreas at operation or at necropsy, and/or by measuring the levels of pancreatic hormones, particularly serum amylase.

Most papers describe hospital in-patient or clinic populations. This may be acceptable for acute pancreatitis, but it is not a satisfactory approach for describing the epidemiology of chronic pancreatitis (Durbec and Sarles, 1978; Bourliere and Sarles, 1989; Hayakawa et al., 1989; Little, 1987; Miyake et al., 1989; Amman et al., 1973 and 1987). Thus the papers which claim to deal with chronic pancreatitis are really studying those patients who have survived an acute pancreatic attack. As far as I have been able to determine, there have been no surveys of pancreatic function in any non-hospital population. One possible exception is a study of pancreatic enzyme levels in drunken drivers (Niederau et al., 1990). This paper claims that, because pancreatic enzymes had weaker correlations than hepatic enzymes with the drivers' alcohol levels, the pancreas is less susceptible to acute injury from alcohol than the liver. Such a conclusion is quite unjustified because it does not consider how the enzyme levels relate to disease severity.

8.4 Diagnostic criteria for acute pancreatitis

The majority of papers in this area are uncontrolled reports of patient series. The criteria for the inclusion of patients in these series, and in other studies, are not always clear. Where a set of diagnostic criteria is given, and inclusion conditions are stated, there are clearly major differences between studies in the definitions used. For example, Thomson et al. (1987) obtained their cases by reviewing all serum samples assayed in the hospital laboratory and investigating cases who had contributed a sample with a level of serum amylase above 1000 iu/l. Cases were accepted into the series if there was a consistent clinical history. Further cases were included in the study because they had pathological evidence of pancreatitis, and it is not clear how many cases were ascertained in these different ways. Different cut-offs for serum amylase have been used in other studies, as have different methods of patient ascertainment. There appears to have been no attempt at any objective classification of this disease. Such criteria might be based on the duration and intensity of pancreatic pain, in combination with serum amylase levels and pathology results. The timing of the serum amylase levels may be important in relation to the duration and intensity of pain (Wyllie and Gunn, 1979).

Given the variation in diagnostic criteria, it is not surprising that those studies which have attempted to estimate the population incidence of acute pancreatitis have obtained a wide variety of results. Schmidt et al. (1991) reviewed hospital admissions in Stockholm over the period 1969–87 and found a trend which peaked in 1974 at a rate of 401 per million. Other estimates have ranged from 242 per million in north-east Scotland (Thomson et al., 1987) to 6 per million in Bristol (Trapnell and Duncan,

1975), with a range of intermediate values. These differences are much more likely to be the result of different definitions of the disease than of any true differences between the populations studied.

A history of biliary disease, such as gallstones, is a common presenting feature of pancreatic disease. The cases which present with this history tend to be older, with a peak in the age group 70–80, whereas the largest number of cases without a history of biliary disease are in the age range 30–60 years (Thomson et al., 1987, and other references). The sex ratio differs according to the history of biliary disease. More women than men present with pancreatitis with a history of biliary disease, whereas the percentage of males is higher in those presenting without such a history.

Most studies of acute pancreatitis have attempted to classify the disease into various categories. The biliary category is one such, and somewhat different criteria have been used to define it. The proportion of patients classified as presenting with biliary disease have ranged from less than 10% (Miyake et al., 1989) to 30% for men and 53% for women (Thomson et al., 1987).

Even less helpful is the classification of non-biliary disease into 'alcoholic' and 'idiopathic'. Different rules have been used in each study for what constitutes 'alcoholic'. For example, Miyake et al. (1989) used the criterion of greater than 85g of alcohol per day over a ten-year period. On this criterion, they classified over 60% of their non-biliary cases as 'alcoholic'. Some studies (e.g. Thomson et al., 1987) have even relied on the mention of alcohol problems in patients' notes as a basis of this classification. The way in which the alcohol consumption data were obtained is never stated.

There seem to be some parallels between non-biliary and biliary pancreatitis, and alcoholic and non-alcoholic cirrhosis (Kreitman and Duffy, 1989). The age and sex distributions for each pair of diseases are similar, with the disease which is presumed not to be alcohol-related occurring more frequently in women and in the older age groups.

There have been various follow-up studies of patients who presented with acute pancreatitis (e.g. McEntee et al., 1987). These show that for 'alcoholic' pancreatitis, there is a high rate of recurrence and repeated hospital admissions and surgery. One study (Hayakawa et al., 1989) also shows that the five-year mortality was greater in those patients classified as 'alcoholic'.

Amman and his colleagues (1973 and 1987) have conducted follow-up studies of patients in Zurich with chronic pancreatitis, the majority of whom were classified as 'alcoholic' on the relatively strict criterion of more than 80g per day of pure ethanol for at least five years. The data are not presented in a manner which allows mortality rates to be calculated. However, the overall death rate in the 1987 study was 40%, for patients with an average age of 43 years followed up for an average of 6.7 years. Only 10 of the 83 deaths in this study were classified as being due to pancreatitis. Other causes were infections (16 cases), malignancy (14 cases), cardiovascular (12 cases) and cirrhosis/hepatitis (9 cases).

8.5 Trends in alcohol consumption and rates of pancreatic disease

Several studies have attempted to relate trends in alcohol consumption over time to trends in admission rates for pancreatic disease. There are several problems with this type of study. The trends in admission rates may reflect trends in the diagnostic criteria used to classify admissions; the proportion of the population consuming very large quantities of alcohol may not follow the same trends as the mean consumption; and time lags may complicate the picture. The study which provides the most convincing evidence is that of Poikolainen et al. (1980), which looked at the period 1968–74 in Finland when a very sharp increase in alcohol consumption occurred in a short time. Admission rates for pancreatic disease increased from 410 to 830 per million per year for men and from 290 to 400 per million per year for women. This was a much steeper increase than was seen in the corresponding figures for liver cirrhosis.

It is also interesting to note that in this study and in the Stockholm study (Schmidt, 1991) admission rates for pancreatitis were roughly twice those for liver cirrhosis. This is in contrast to the mortality figures, which show that liver cirrhosis is a much commoner cause of death than pancreatitis.

8.6 Risks of pancreatitis in relation to alcohol intake

I have only been able to find one acceptable case-control study of alcohol as a risk factor for chronic pancreatitis. This is the study of Durbec and Sarles (1978), which reported a multi-centre case-control study of men from France (the majority of cases), South Africa, Germany, Italy and Denmark. Few details of the cases are given, except that they had a diagnosis of acute pancreatitis, which was identified following an acute attack. It is not clear whether biliary cases are excluded. Controls were taken from the same clinics, with exclusion criteria which included any evidence of cirrhosis of the liver. It is not clear whether this exclusion criterion was also applied to the cases, but the supposition must be that it was not, which may have resulted in a serious overestimation of the risk of pancreatitis from alcohol consumption. Alcohol consumption appears to have been estimated in a similar manner, by questionnaire, for cases and controls.

The results from this study were most striking, and were consistent in the different centres. They show a linear relationship between alcohol consumption and the logarithm of the relative risk of pancreatitis. The risk relative to abstinence rises to around 12 for the category of 80–100g per day, and to around 400 for the highest alcohol category (260–280g per day). There is clear evidence of an increased risk of pancreatitis at levels below 85g/day, which would not be classified as 'alcoholic' in some of the series discussed above.

The contribution of alcohol consumption to pancreatitis mortality is difficult to estimate because of the deficiencies of the research reports which are available in this field. The data in Table 8.1 may not be the full extent of the problem. Amman et al. (1987) showed that the deaths of patients with pancreatitis are often classified as being due to other causes which may be related to the disease. Also, pancreatitis is often associated with diabetes, and one prospective study of chronic pancreatitis (Miyake et al., 1989) has shown that a proportion of deaths of pancreatitis patients may be due to conditions associated with diabetes, such as renal failure. For the purpose of this review, however, we can assume that such deaths would be considered along with the other causes rather than with gastrointestinal disease.

Returning to the mortality data, the case-control data of Durbec and Sarles (1978) would attribute the majority of the deaths due to pancreatitis to alcohol ingestion. However, because of the uncertainty of diagnosis, we cannot be sure that the deaths due to pancreatitis, as coded by the GRO and OPCS, are from a similar population to that studied by Durbec and Sarles. The age and sex distribution of the death rates (lower female mortality at younger ages) would suggest that those cases in the older age groups may not be directly associated with alcohol. However, there is no direct evidence to support this. Alcohol may also play a part in the aetiology of biliary pancreatitis, and females may become susceptible at an older age range. Thus, the best we can suggest is that Table 8.1 gives an upper limit to the mortality from pancreatic disease which is attributable to alcohol consumption in England, Wales and Scotland.

References

Amman, R.W., Buchier, H., Muench, R. and Freiburghaus, A.W. (1987) Differences in natural history of idiopathic (non-alcoholic) and alcoholic chronic pancreatitis, *Pancreas* 2: 368–77.

Amman, R.W., Hammer, B. and Fumagalli, I. (1973) Chronic pancreatitis in Zurich, 1963–72, *Digestion* 9: 404–15.

Bourliere, M. and Sarles, H. (1989) Pancreatic cysts and pseudocysts associated with acute and chronic pancreatitis, *Digestive Diseases and Sciences* 34: 343–8.

Durbec, J.P. and Sarles, H. (1978) Multicenter survey of the etiology of pancreatic disease, *Digestion* 18: 337–50.

Hayakawa, T., Kondo, T., Shibata, T., Sugimoto, Y. and Kitagawa, M. (1989) Chronic alcoholism and evolution of pain and prognosis in chronic pancreatitis, *Digestive Diseases and Sciences* 34: 33–8.

Kreitman, N. and Duffy, J. (1989) Alcoholic and non-alcoholic liver disease in relation to alcohol consumption in Scotland, *British Journal of Addiction* 84: 607–18.

Laine, L. (1988) Histology of alcoholic haemorrhagic gastritis: a prospective evaluation, *Gastroenterology* 94: 1254–62.

Little, J.M. (1987) Alcohol abuse and chronic pancreatitis, *Surgery* 101: 357–60.

McEntee, G.P., Gillen, P. and Peel, A.L. (1987) Alcohol induced pancreatitis: social and surgical aspects, *British Journal of Surgery* 74: 402–4.

Miyake, H., Harada, H., Ochi, K., Kunichika, K., Tanaka, J. and Kimura, I. (1989)

Prognosis and prognostic factors in chronic pancreatitis, *Digestive Diseases and Sciences* 34: 449–55.

Naisry, R.W., McIntosh, J.H., Byth, K. and Piper, D.W. (1987) Prognosis of chronic duodenal ulcer: a prospective study of the effects of demographic and environmental factors in ulcer healing, *Gut* 28: 533–40.

Niederau, C., Niederau, M., Strohmeyer, G., Bertling, L. and Sonnenberg, A. (1990) Does acute consumption of large alcohol amounts lead to pancreatic injury? *Digestion* 45: 115–20.

Poikolainen, K. (1980) Increase in alcohol-related hospital admissions in Finland (1969–75), *British Journal of Addiction* 75: 281–91.

Reynolds, J.C. (1989) Pamotidine therapy for active duodenal ulcers. A multivariate analysis of factors affecting early healing, *Annals of Internal Medicine* 111: 7–14.

Sarles, H., Bernard, J.P. and Johnson, C. (1989) Pathogenesis and epidemiology of chronic pancreatitis, *Annual Review of Medicine* 40: 453–68.

Segawa, K., Nakazawa, S., Tsukamoto, Y., Goto, H., Yamao, K., Hase, S., Osada, T. and Arisawa, T. (1988) Chronic alcohol abuse leads to gastric atrophy and decreased gastric secretory capacity: a histological and physiological study, *American Journal of Gastroenterology* 83: 373–9.

Schmidt, D.N. (1991) Apparent risk factors for chronic and acute pancreatitis in Stockholm county, *International Journal of Pancreatology* 8: 45–50.

Thomson, S.R., Hendry, W.S., McFarlane, G.A. and Davidson, A.I. (1987) Epidemiology and outcome of acute pancreatitis, *British Journal of Surgery* 74: 398–401.

Trapnell, J.E. and Duncan, E.H. (1975) Patterns of incidence in acute pancreatitis, *British Medical Journal* 2: 179–83.

Walker, P., Luther, J., Samloff, M. and Feldman, M. (1988) Life events stress and psychological factors in men with peptic ulcer disease, *Gastroenterology* 94: 323–30.

Wyllie, F.J. and Gunn, A.A. (1979) Diagnosis of acute pancreatitis, *Journal of the Royal College of Surgeons of Edinburgh* 24: 363–7.

9 Conclusion – Other Aspects of Alcohol and Harm

The preceding chapters have summarised current epidemiological knowledge and research concerning the relationship between alcohol consumption and physical illness. There are clearly other areas in which the consumption of alcohol may be associated with the development of problems, notably accidents, crime, psychiatric illness, employment and interpersonal relations. In each of these, there are considerable difficulties of estimating the possible causal contribution of alcohol consumption.

At the same time, for reasons of public policy formation, there is considerable pressure on researchers to produce estimates of quantities such as 'total mortality due to alcohol consumption', 'life years lost due to alcohol consumption', 'cost to society of alcohol-related problems and damage' and so on. As mentioned in Chapter 3, McDonnell and Maynard (1985) attempted to estimate total mortality attributable to alcohol abuse, and elaborated this to estimate 'life years lost' from alcohol-related premature death. It is not intended to go into the details of the calculations used here, but instead to note that, for the various causes considered, attributable mortality from a specified cause was assumed to be the same in all age groups. This is a highly unlikely contingency, given the known differences in consumption between ages, quite apart from possible differences in the relation between alcohol consumption and risk which may exist at different ages.

For this reason, there has been no attempt in this work to produce estimates of years of life lost. In most cases, too, the authors have not attempted to produce estimates of total mortality attributable to alcohol, but have confined themselves to estimation in specified subgroups of the population (e.g. middle-aged men) for which data are available to estimate risk relationships. Of course, if studies concern all age groups in the population of interest, then it is appropriate to use the information contained in these to estimate total attributable mortality.

9.1 Accidents

Road accident deaths are an obvious source of mortality possibly attributable to alcohol. In 1988, the Department of Transport (1990) estimated that 840 fatalities occurred in drink-drive accidents, that is accidents in which at least one driver or rider failed a breath test, or at least one driver or rider who was killed had a blood alcohol level above the legal limit. There are obvious problems of under-reporting, from breath-testing not being carried out at the time of the accident or within twelve hours following the accident. Even adjusting for these, there still remains the problem of attribution of the accident to alcohol consumption. It is not beyond the bounds of possibility that some of these accidents may have occurred even though no driver or rider involved in them had consumed alcohol. At the same time, some of the accidents in which no driver or rider was over the legal limit may have been due to the reduction in driving skills known to take place in susceptible individuals at blood alcohol levels below the legal limit. A forthcoming report from the Transport and Road Research Laboratory (in press) indicates that around 14% of all road casualties attending accident and emergency departments had been drinking, which sets an upper limit on the proportion of such casualties which might be alcohol-related.

Alcohol is likely to play a part in accidents of other kinds, such as industrial accidents, domestic accidents, fires, accidental poisonings and drownings. However, there appear to be few studies which would permit estimation of the proportion of these attributable to alcohol. This has not deterred some authorities from producing 'guesstimates' in this area, notably the Royal College of General Practitioners (1986), who attribute 40% of all deaths due to injuries and poisonings in both sexes to alcohol, which compares strangely with McDonnell and Maynard's earlier 'high' estimates of 33% for men and 6% for women. A more recent investigation (Chick et al., 1991) suggests that a proportion of around 19% of male admissions to an acute orthopaedic ward were alcohol-related, although there are some deficiencies in the methods of analysis employed.

9.2 Crime

Restricting attention to alcohol and crime-related mortality, there were 164 male and 113 female deaths officially recorded as due to homicide or deliberately-inflicted injury by another person in England and Wales in 1989 (OPCS, 1991). Even if there is a considerable element of undercounting, it is clear that crime-related mortality is not a major cause of death and will contribute little to any estimate of total mortality attributable to alcohol.

9.3 Psychiatric illness

Psychiatric morbidity and mortality explicitly recorded as due to alcohol are unlikely to be an adequate representation of the contribution of alcohol to such conditions. Admissions to mental hospitals for alcoholism, alcohol dependence syndrome or related conditions in different regions of the country have been found to reflect medical policy rather than real differences (Crawford et al., 1985). Thus, the decline in psychiatric hospital admissions with alcohol diagnoses noted by Duffy and Plant (1986) was not considered by them to be an accurate reflection of the level of psychiatric problems associated with alcohol misuse.

Explicitly psychiatric mortality associated with alcohol is rare. In England and Wales in 1989, 10 deaths were attributed to alcoholic psychoses, 148 to the alcohol dependence syndrome and 124 to alcohol (OPCS, 1991). Alcoholism is known to increase the risk of suicide (Murphy and Wetzel, 1990), and, for epidemiological purposes, deaths officially recorded as undetermined may be aggregated with suicide deaths, on the grounds that many of these would be classed as suicide on psychiatric, although not on legal, criteria (Ovenstone, 1973). Overall, there were 3,717 deaths by suicide and self-inflicted injury in England and Wales in 1989, and a further 1,986 deaths by injury undetermined as to whether accidentally or purposely inflicted. Clearly, if the proportion of these deaths related to alcohol is large, this could constitute an important source of alcohol-related mortality.

9.4 Economic considerations

Attempts to establish the costs to society of alcohol consumption are not uncommon, in the form of calculations of revenues (for example, excise taxation) and costs to the state of dealing with the effects of consumption. The private costs and benefits to the individual are generally left out of account, while the public or social costs are based on estimates of the various forms of social and health damage resulting from consumption. On this basis, for example, Walsh (1990) concludes that in the United Kingdom 'the drinker pays his way', although he includes only public sector costs in his analysis.

Most of these estimates of social costs are of unknown accuracy, and, as pointed out by Maynard (1989), the empirical basis of such estimation has improved little in recent years. A selection of the following may be found on the debit side of the account: costs to industry incurred through absenteeism, illness and premature death; costs to the National Health Service of treatment of alcohol-attributed episodes of illness; research and educational expenditure; material damage and crime related costs. On the credit side, it is usual to find only one item, the yield of special taxes related to alcohol.

The problems in costing the contribution of alcohol to ill health should be clear after reading the earlier chapters of this volume. If it is difficult to estimate attributable mortality from a particular condition, it is in general even more difficult to estimate attributable morbidity, and to attempt to do so for all conditions treated by the National Health Service is optimistic indeed. Chapter 3 also makes clear the implications of the possible protective effect of moderate consumption of alcohol on heart disease. If the protective effect really exists, then far from years of life lost being costed and set down as a debit in the account, it would be appropriate to estimate years of life gained, and set the financial value of these on the credit side.

In fact, the appropriateness of any such calculation is seriously questionable. Maynard (1989) summarises the deficiencies in the approach as follows:

- the cost and health estimates are poor because of the inadequate epidemiological and economic bases from which they are derived;
- the benefits to the user of alcohol use are ignored;
- the policy-relevant data are about the margin, not the total or average.

The last point emphasises that estimating total costs or benefits to society is essentially inadequate as a guide to action. Estimates of the effects of policy interventions on the quantities on either side of the account are of much more importance, but in the present state of knowledge are extremely difficult to produce.

References

Chick, J., Rund, D. and Gilbert, M.-A. (1991) Orthopaedic trauma in men: the relative risk among drinkers and the prevalence of problem drinking in male orthopaedic admissions, *Annals of the Royal College of Surgeons of England* 73: 311–15.

Crawford, A., Plant, M.A., Kreitman, N. and Latcham, R.W. (1985) Self-reported alcohol consumption and adverse consequences of drinking in three areas of Britain: general population studies, *British Journal of Addiction* 80: 421–8.

Department of Transport (1990) *Accident Fact Sheet 3/90*, London: HMSO.

Duffy, J.C. and Plant, M.A. (1986) Scotland's liquor licensing changes: an assessment, *British Medical Journal* 292: 36–9.

Maynard, A. (1989) The costs of addiction and the costs of control, in Robinson, D., Maynard, A. and Chester, R. (eds) *Controlling Legal Addictions*, London: Macmillan.

McDonnell, R. and Maynard, A. (1985) Estimation of life-years lost from alcohol-related premature death, *Alcohol and Alcoholism* 20: 435–43.

Murphy, G. and Wetzel, R. (1990) The lifetime risk of suicide in alcoholism, *Archives of General Psychiatry* 47: 383–92.

Office of Population Censuses and Surveys (1991) *1989 Mortality Statistics: Cause*, London: HMSO.

Ovenstone, I. (1973) A psychiatric approach to the diagnosis of suicide and its effect in the Edinburgh statistics, *British Journal of Psychiatry* 123: 15–22.

Royal College of General Practitioners (1986) *Alcohol: a Balanced View*, London: RCGP.

Transport and Road Research Laboratory (in press) *Research Report 311*, Crowthorne: TRRL.

Walsh, B.M. (1990) *Alcohol, the Economy and Public Health*, Copenhagen: World Health Organisation Regional Office for Europe.

Index